Healthy
LIVING
SPACES

Top 10 Hazards
Affecting
Your Health

Daniel Stih

BSE, CMC, CIEC

D0815157

Layout and cover design by John Cole.
Cover image by John Mate.

ISBN 13: 978-097946850-6
ISBN 10: 097946850-7

Inquiries regarding requests to reprint all or part of
Healthy Living Spaces should be addressed to the
publisher at the address below:

Healthy Living Spaces
369 Montezuma Ave #169
Santa Fe, NM 87501

DISCLAIMER

This book is designed for educational purposes only.

Our goal is to provide information and scientific data as to the potential hazards in the home or office. All the factors to be considerd are beyond the scope of this book. We do not assume responsibility for choices or decisions made including those regarding mitigation. The principles presented here should empower the reader to make informed choices. If in doubt, consult a professional.

This book is not intended to provide medical or legal advice. The services of a competent professional should be obtained whenever medical, legal or other specific advice is needed.

The listing of any particular product is not an endorsement of that product. The reader is encouraged to do their own research to supplement information that is provided here before making choices.

ACKNOWLEDGEMENTS

I got into this business after retiring as an engineer and becoming a handyman. I would often come home covered in paint and toxic dust from a variety of sources. My partner at the time put a bug in my ear that the chemicals were being absorbed into my body though my skin. That started me on this path.

Many thanks to the staff at the Institute for Building Biology, including Will Spates, Lawrence Gust and Spark Burmaster, for a wealth of information always generously given.

Paul Baker-Laporte for her support and suggestions for getting a book written and published.

My editor, Cynthia Green at THEMA, Ideas in Print. Where other editors could not see the forest through the trees of my original manuscript, Cynthia suggested the simplified format of the book you are reading now.

Megan Kemple of the Northwest Coalition for Alternatives to Pesticides (NCAP) and Elizabeth Guillette, Ph.D. for reviewing the chapter on Pesticides; Karl Riley for reviewing the chapter on Electromagnetic Fields.

Thanks to my parents for their love and support.

Other individuals have provided support and information. I thank them all.

The endnotes are dedicated to my brother John, the skeptic.

TABLE OF CONTENTS

INTRODUCTION

My Home or Office Unhealthy?

The teepee is much better to live in; always clean, warm in winter, cool in summer, easy to move. The white man builds big house, cost much money, like big cage, shut sun out, can never move; always sick... Indians and animals know better how to live... Nobody can be in good health if he does not have all the time fresh air, sunshine and good water...

— Chief Flying Hawk, Ogalala Sioux, nephew of Sitting Bull[1]

We tend to think of our homes as safe havens, places that protect and nurture us. We may not like going to the office, but we typically do not think of the office as toxic. Unfortunately, the Environmental Protection Agency estimates that pollution indoors can be six to ten times higher than outside and is responsible for serious health effects. Because we spend 90% of our time indoors, we are potentially exposed to 90% of the factors that cause illness while we are indoors. The indoors is widely recognized as one of the most serious risks to human health.

You don't have to live in an unhealthy home or office. This book provides you with a roadmap to identifying the worst offenders and correcting them. In today's world it seems everything is thought to cause cancer or be bad for your health. But most homes and offices typically have only a few environmental factors that are responsible for the bulk of potential harm. This book contains a list of the Top Ten. It is based on the investigation of hundreds of homes, offices, and schools.

You can't worry about everything. I am suggesting that 90% of health complaints related to the indoors are due to 10% of the infinite number of hazards we are exposed to. What will your state of health and well-being look like when these are gone?

How to Use this book

Your immediate reaction after picking up this book may be to skim the chapter titles and see if anything jumps out. That may be a good idea. If you think you have a mold problem or smell mold, start with mold. The National Institute for Occupations Safety and Health suggests that 35% to 50% of all *Sick Building* cases are due to mold.

Mold is often not the problem, or there may be another hazard working in synergy with mold to acerbate the effect it is having on your health. For example, I often show up at people's homes to do a mold inspection and can't smell the mold because of the plug-in air fresheners or mothballs. Ironically, the occupants have gotten so used to the smell of the fragrance and chemicals they can't smell them. It often turns out that mold is not their problem but the level of fragrance and pesticides from the mothballs is causing them great harm.

The heating and air conditioning systems are often contaminated and responsible for complaints, especially in large office buildings. Simply giving it a check-up and cleaning it can make everyone in the building happier. This is covered in a few sections including Mystery Toxins.

Determining exactly what is causing toxicity in your indoor world can be a puzzle. But it is not rocket science. This simple guide can radically improve the health of your living space.

The Rain Barrel Effect

To you, it may not seem like any single item on the Top 10 list is affecting your health. Studies that indicate the items on the list play a role in the creation of allergies and illness show that no single factor causes illness. Rather, the cumulative load of multiple poisons creates allergies and illness. People don't get disease, they *develop* it.[2]

Picture an empty barrel outside in the rain. A few raindrops in the bottom of an empty barrel are not noticed. Left out in the rain long enough, however, and one more drop will make the barrel overflow. It is the straw that breaks the camel's back, so to speak. It's the same thing with the body's immune system. It can only handle so much. Toxic mold may cause the body to have an allergic reaction. But it is the dust, cleaning products, fragrance, pesticides, new carpet, fresh paint, and sleeping next to the TV that made the body vulnerable to mold.

It takes two to tango. Not only do combinations of several toxins weaken the immune system, certain pairs are especially interactive. Researchers have found a synergistic effect between tobacco smoke and mold; tobacco smoke and allergens in house dust; mold and pet dog dander.[3]

There is also a relationship between exterior and interior allergens. If you are allergic to pollen, cleaning up your indoor environment may not eliminate your allergies. But it may help. By reducing the load on your immune system from other pollutants you may find your body more able to resist your other sensitivities. There are suggestions in this book that can be used to pollen proof your home. (See bringing in HEPA filtered outdoor air in furnace filter recommendations).

After you look over the Top Ten list, you will have a good concept of the major problem areas and how to address them. You will also be able to look at the bigger picture of interacting and cumulative irritants and know how to cleanse your living space for a gentler, safer environment.

END NOTES

1. Coppinger, Joyce. "Natural Ventilation: let there be air, fresh air." *The Last Straw* #48. Winter, 2005, p. 12.
2. Kail, Konrad, N.D. and Bobbi Lawrence. *Allergy Free, An Alternative Medicine Definitive Guide.* AlterntiveMedicine.com, 2000, p. 58.
3. Wiles. Charlie. *Certified Microbial Consultant Review Course.* The American Indoor Air Quality Council, 2003. See also: Alfred V. Zamm, M.D., *Why Your House May Endanger Your Health.* Simon and Shuster, 1980, pp. 34, 37.

1 : Mold

WHAT IS IT?

Mold, mildew, and fungus all refer to the same thing. Molds are the garbage men of the universe. It is mold's job to break things down. Otherwise the earth would be piled sky-high in rubbish. If something gets wet and stays wet, mold will grow, not matter how hard you try and stop it. The only way to prevent mold growth is to keep things dry. Period.

Mold has a tough outer shell that protects it from sunlight and ultraviolet light. It can survive thousands of years, waiting for water.

The bulk of mold growth consists of a mass of branches called *hyphae*. The branches are similar to branches on a tree. Mold spores are attached to the end of the branches, like seeds.

Curvularia mold spores attached to a mass of hyphae (branches). Courtesy Environmental Microbiology Laboratory, Inc.

WHAT CAN IT DO TO ME?

Allergic response and cold and flu-like symptoms are the most common health symptoms associated with mold exposure. People often ask how many mold spores it takes to make them sick. A single spore of pollen may be enough for someone allergic to pollen to have a reaction; the same may be true for certain species of mold.

All molds are allergenic and potentially toxigenic.[1] Your response depends on your immune system, the dose, and the duration of exposure. Dead mold spores are still allergenic and potentially toxic. Allergens and toxins are not neutralized with bleach or other chemicals. Therefore, dead or alive, mold can cause allergic reactions in people.[2] For mold remediation to be effective, mold needs to be physically removed, not just "killed."

Symptoms of Mold Exposure

- Allergies and Irritation

- Cold and Flu symptoms

- Burning, itchy eyes and skin

- Difficulty breathing

- Dry, hacking cough, sore throat

- Headaches

- Nosebleeds

- Fatigue

Molds produce chemicals from normal metabolism and digesting foods. Some of the chemicals produced are similar to those in paint and nail polish. Some cause musty odors. They are irritants and toxic to the nervous system. They may cause headache, inability to concentrate, nausea, foggy thinking, and respiratory problems.

Mold can suppress the immune system.[3] The longer someone is exposed to mold, the more likely they are to be affected and the more severe the symptoms may be. Chronic exposure may lead to the development of allergies or asthma in otherwise healthy people.

Fortunately most people, if they have not occupied a mold-contaminated environment for very long, recover after they move out or the mold is cleaned up.

WHERE IS IT?

Mold can grow anywhere, on nearly anything, and is hiding fifty percent of the time. There are even mold problems in dry Phoenix, Arizona, in the summer, the driest time of year.

Plumbing leaks are the #1 cause for mold growth. Nearly every modern building has indoor plumbing. It doesn't matter if your home is new or old: if building materials inside your home get wet and don't dry out fast enough, mold will grow. The first 48 hours are the most critical. Mold starts to grow within 24 hours. After 48 hours the probability of contamination is likely if things are still wet.

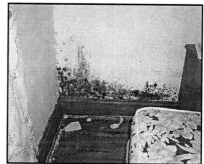

Mold on a bedroom wall due to condensation. There was too much humidity in the room and the wall was cold because warm air could not get to it. Courtesy Martine Davis, Environmental Testing Inc.

Mold likes dampness. Find the damp spot and you will often find the mold. It is useful to have a moisture meter when checking for dampness (see the Resource section at the end of this chapter). Surfaces may look dry when they are actually damp. Look for mold and dampness in the following places:

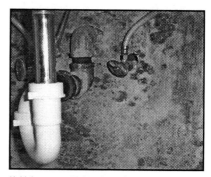

Mold is commonly found growing under kitchen sinks. If it smells musty under the kitchen sink look for mold.

- Under kitchen & bathroom sinks

- Around hot water heaters

- Behind washing machines and dishwashers

- Behind the toilet near the water shut-off valve

- Under carpeting that has become wet

- Behind and under boxes and personal contents stored in closets

- Crawlspaces and attics

- Air-conditioning drain pans and filters

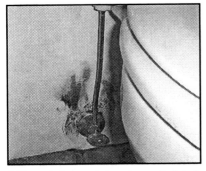

Mold growth due to a leaky water supply shut-off valve behind the toilet.

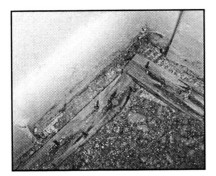

If you are buying a house, pull back carpet under windows or near exterior doors. Discolored, rusty carpet tacks are a sign of water intrusion. It may be from either a flood, leaving the windows open or a leak inside the wall.

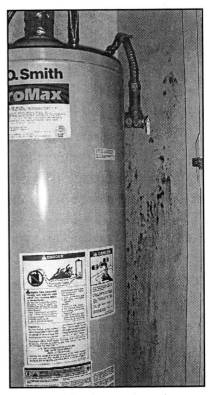

Mold on a wall in a hot water heater closet.

TESTING FOR MOLD

If you want to test your home for mold, hire a professional. Many people who test their homes using self-test kits end up confused by the results. They may think they have a mold problem when they don't, or that their home is safe when there is in fact a mold problem.

The primary problem with self-test kits is that they use petri dishes as settling plates. Heavier mold spores settle out of the air faster than lighter ones, skewing

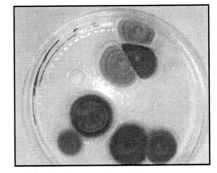

Petri dish used to test for mold.

the results. Less than 2% of mold spores will grow in a petri dish. Those that do will compete for survival. What is in the air may not be what wins the battle in the petri dish.

GET RID OF IT!!!

If mold has grown into porous building materials like drywall, the wall must be cut out. Drywall contaminated with mold cannot be cleaned. If the mold is on a hard surface such as wood, glass, or metal, it can be cleaned.

The first thing to consider when cleaning up mold is the size of contamination. There is going to be a different approach to cleaning mildew off your shower than mold growing inside walls. There are some government guidelines for determining what level of training is required to clean up mold based on how many square feet of mold is visible. These guidelines can be misleading. When you see a few square inches of mold growth on a wall there is typically much more hidden inside the wall.

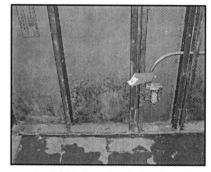

Stachybotrys mold inside a wall. There is usually a lot more hidden mold inside a wall than is visible on the front side.

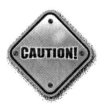

CAN YOU DO IT YOURSELF?

As with any activity there is a learning curve. You usually don't do everything right the first time around. Removing mold from your home or office may be a job better left for a professional. There are techniques to minimize dispersal of mold spores and to protect yourself and workers. This may or may not be a huge issue depending on the amount of mold present and the sensitivities of the occupants.

Sometimes all these precautions seem to be over-kill. Mold is not the bubonic plague. At other times, careless work has resulted in the occupants forever being affected by allergies due to small levels of mold spores that were distributed throughout the house.

See the resource section at the end of this chapter to find a certified consultant or professional mold remediator.

INTERIM RELIEF

If it's going to be a while before you can clean up the mold there are some things you should do to contain the mold and protect your health:

- Do not run the air conditioner or forced air heating.

- If it is a small area, carefully cover the mold with plastic. Cut up a trash bag and secure it with duck-tape over the mold, being very careful to not disturb the mold. The self adhesive plastic that is used to cover and protect carpet is useful. It can be found at most hardware stores.

- Close the door to the room mold is in and avoid going into that room.

- Use a *high efficiency particulate air* [HEPA] purifier in the room where you spend most of your time.

WHAT NOT TO DO

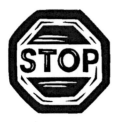

Do not use bleach. Bleach does not kill mold.[4]

Do not disturb mold until you have an action plan that considers containment and personal protection.

Do not use ozone. Ozone does not kill mold. Ozone is a respiratory irritant that has been found to scar lungs in lab rats.[5]

Do not paint over mold. Paint is food for mold. Mold will grow through paint, even paint that contains ingredients to prohibit mold.

Do not use fans. Fans will blow mold around. If things are wet you should remove the mold before using a fan to dry things out.

WHAT TO DO

Notice: It is outside the scope of this book to plan for all the potential variables that may be encountered during mold remediation work. The following is not intended to imply or express any guarantee regarding effective remediation of mold, protection of workers, and prevention of cross-contamination.

Protect yourself. Do not clean up mold if you have allergies or sensitivities. Wear a half-face or full-face respirator with a HEPA filter cartridge (P100), goggles, disposable gloves, and disposable coveralls or a Tyvek suit.

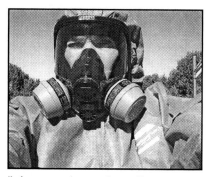
You've got to take care of yourself.

Contain the dust. Use methods that contain the dust and mold spores. Where there may have been only a few mold spores in the air prior to cleaning, trillions of unseen mold spores are aerosolized during mold remediation. Cover all contents, furniture, cabinets, closets, book shelves, drapes, etc. with plastic secured with duct tape. Hang plastic over the doorway to isolate the room where the work is being done from the rest of the house. Cover floors with plastic unless the carpet will be removed. Shut down the heating and cooling system. Seal furnace supply and return air conditioning and heating vents. Do not run the heating or air-conditioning system while work is being done.

Professionals use air scrubbers that exhaust air from the work area to the outdoors, creating a vacuum in the room they are working in relative to the rest of the house. During demolition the dust generated is sucked into the air scrubber and kept from contaminating the rest of the house.

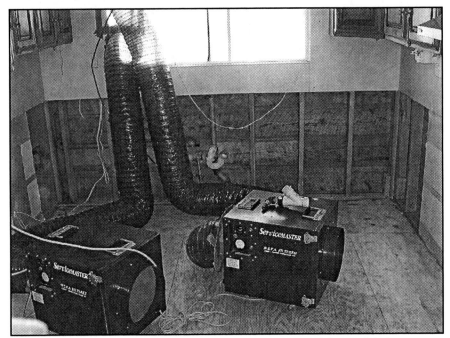

Air scrubbers are used to suck dust up, keeping it as well as mold spores out of the rest of the house.

Carefully remove mold. Moldy materials should be removed carefully so as not to agitate mold or generate dust. Use a razor instead of a saw to cut drywall. Remove drywall, particleboard, and insulation at least two feet beyond where mold growth is visible. Carpet and padding that has visible mold growth should be discarded.

Place materials in heavy duty trash bags. There are no special requirements for the disposal. You can just throw mold out with regular trash. It will be a crazy day if mold becomes regulated waste. Every compost pile on the farm will become a hazardous waste site!

Sand and wire-brush. If necessary, wire-brush or sand the wood, plywood, and concrete block while keeping a HEPA vacuum nearby to capture the dust. Rot should be removed. Wood does not have to be sanded until there is no staining present. The dark stains on wood are due to enzymes. Since molds don't have stomachs, they secret enzymes onto materials to digest them. These enzymes are responsible for the dark staining that accompanies mold growth. Mold only grows a short distance into wood. The remainder of the stain is simply a stain.

Clean. After all moldy building materials have been removed, clean the remaining surfaces. Do not use cleaning methods that raise dust such as sweeping with brooms. Use a HEPA vacuum. Some people place a shop vacuum outdoors and put the hose through a window to vacuum indoors.

Use what ever you would normally use to clean a dirty surface. Plain soap and water will do. Bleach and chemicals are not necessary. If the mold is effectively removed there should be nothing left to kill. Clean rags should be folded in quarters. Ring the rag out after dipping it in soapy water. Make only one pass over a surface, then flip the rag over and use a clean side.

Cleaning requires careful attention to detail and a diligence that may be difficult to appreciate since you can't see microscopic mold spores. Vacuuming itself does not clean fine dust. Mold spores cling to surfaces electro-statically. Do a white-glove test. You should be able to eat off the floor when you are finished.

If you feel the need to use an antimicrobial, even though there shouldn't be any mold spores left to kill, here are some alternatives:

- Dr. Bronner's Peppermint soap

- Vinegar (1/4 cup to 1 gallon of water)

- Hydrogen peroxide (3%)

- Borax. Make a paste with water to scrub with.

Clean your stuff. Don't throw all your stuff away just because it was stored inside a building with mold. If your belongings did not have mold growing on them but were simply in close proximity to mold, they may be cleaned by HEPA vacuuming, regular laundering, or dry cleaning. It also works to take them outside and beat them like a rug.

Consider throwing away porous personal belongings such as clothing, carpet, and upholstered furniture that are contaminated with visible mold growth. It can be difficult to effectively remove active mold growth by cleaning. An odor may remain even after the mold is gone.

Clean hard contents such as wood furniture by HEPA vacuuming and damp wiping using plain soap and water. If mold grew on wood furniture it can be sanded off. Take the furniture outside. Wear a respirator.

Prevent mold from coming back.
Water it and they will grow! The cause of the moisture must be identified and eliminated otherwise mold will grow back. Fix that plumbing or roof leak. If necessary ventilate the attic or crawl-space better. Don't rebuild until things have dried out.

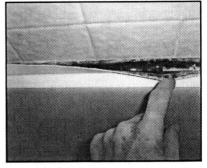

Mold growth behind trim around a bath tub. Keep the edge around the tub caulked and tile cracks grouted to prevent water from getting behind them.

NANA'S KITCHEN

One of my first experiences with mold was a project I did for my grandmother, Nana. She is 90 years old. She wanted to give her house a real, old-fashioned cleaning, where you wipe the walls down from floor to ceiling. She didn't trust anyone else to do a good job so I told her I would do it.

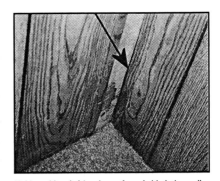

Mold peeking its' head out from behind the wall paneling.

While I was wiping down the walls, I noticed a small, black, vertical line in a corner on a wall between the kitchen and living room. The décor was fake wood paneling. From a distance the line looked one of the groves that are etched into wood paneling.

To investigate further, I poked my head under the kitchen sink and pulled back the paneling between the kitchen cabinet and the wall. There was an incredible amount of mold hiding there. The pipes

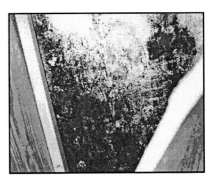

Who would have thought so much mold could be present when almost none was visible before the paneling was pulled back.

under the kitchen sink had leaked before Nana bought her house. Things were dry now, but there was a lot of mold behind all of the walls in the kitchen.

The cost to hire a professional mold remediator to clean up the mold would run thousands of dollars. To save Nana money, I told her I would clean up the mold. I bought an air-scrubber and HEPA vacuum and commenced to remove the mold from her kitchen.

Nearly all of the walls in the kitchen had mold behind them and needed to be removed. There was mold hiding in places no one ever looks including behind the range and refrigerator. I tore out the built-in cabinets and there was mold on the walls behind them.

When I was done tearing out all the walls, everything looked clean, but I could still smell something coming from under the floor. To investigate, I cut a small hole in the floor large enough to peek my head under. There was mold on the underside of the entire kitchen floor. The whole floor needed to be removed.

I learned two lessons learned from this. First, when you see a little bit of mold, a lot may be hiding. The only visible sign of mold here had been that tiny black streak which was overlooked, perhaps hidden by the TV set. Second, the job's not done until the odor is gone.

I finished cleaning and Nana's kitchen was rebuilt. The next time I stopped by to see her, I noticed that I felt different being in her home. Previously something had not felt right, but I couldn't put my finger on it. Even Nana seemed to be a more mentally alert. She had been getting some comments about having Alzheimer's, but I now found her to be sharp as a tack.

RESOURCES

Healthy Living Spaces
Visit the website: HealthyLivingSpaces.com
Call: toll-free (877) 992-9904, (505) 992-9904
Your one-stop for mold abatement equipment, protective gear, respirators, vacuum cleaners, and the S520 Mold Guide

The Yellow Pages
If you have a sudden flood, plumbing, or roof leak, call a professional immediately. Look in the yellow pages under *Water Damage Restoration*. DO NOT wait for an insurance adjuster to visit you house. The clock is ticking.

Moisture Meters
Professional Equipment
Phone: (800) 334-9291
Web site: www.professionalequipment.com
The Survey Master by Protimeter is recommended

Respirators, goggles, gloves, and Tyvek™ suits
Lab Safety
Phone: (800) 356-0783
Web site: www.labsafety.com.

Professional Equipment
Phone: (800) 334-9291
Web site: www.professionalequipment.com

Air Scrubbers
Abatement Technologies
Phone: (800) 634-9091
Web site: www.abatement.com

HEPA Vacuums
Miele
Phone: (800) 843-7231
Web site: www.miele.com

Nilfisk
Phone: (610) 647 6420
Web sites: http://nilfisk.com and www.pa.nilfisk-advance.com

To find a Certified Mold Inspector (Microbial Consultant or Mold Remediator)
The American Indoor Air Quality Council
Phone: (800) 942-0832
Web site: www.iaqcouncil.org

Asbestos and Lead Paint
Buildings constructed before 1977 and as late as 1983 may contain asbestos. It is commonly found on furnace pipe insulation, pop-corn ceilings, vinyl floor tile, wall board and textured paint. Buildings constructed before 1960 and as late as 1978 may contain lead paint. Usually the same environmental testing companies that do testing for mold can do testing for lead paint and asbestos. For information on lead paint and asbestos, visit: www.epa.gov/lead or www.epa.gov/asbestos

For Education and Training
The Indoor Air Quality Association
Phone: (301) 231-8388
Web site: www.iaqa.org

SUGGESTED READING

IICRC S520 Standard and Reference Guide for Professional Mold Remediation.
IICRC S500 Standard and Reference Guide for Professional water Damage Restoration.
Order from the Indoor Air Quality Association (IAQA). Phone: (301) 231-8388.
Web site: www.iaqa.org.

EPA documents may be viewed or down-loaded on-line at http://www.epa.gov/mold.
Hard-copies can be ordered on-line or by calling (800) 438-4318 or (703) 356-4020.

A Brief Guide to Mold, Moisture and Your Home, EPA 402-K-02-003.

Mold Remediation in Schools and Commercial Buildings, EPA 402-K-01-001.

The EPA on-line Mold Course: Introduction to Mold and Mold Remediation for Environmental and Public Health Professionals. www.epa.gov/mdd/moldcourse

END NOTES

1. American Industrial Hygiene Association. *Field Guide for the Determination of Biological Contaminates in Environmental Samples.* American Industrial Hygiene Association, 1996, p. 10.

2. The Environmental Protection Agency. "Chapter 1: Introduction to Mold; Lesson 3: Health Effects That May Be Caused by Inhaling Mold or Mold Spores." *Online Mold Course.* http://www. epa.gov/mold/moldcourse/chapter1/lesson3.html (February 2007). "Mold does not have to be alive to cause an allergic reaction. Dead or alive, mold can cause allergic reactions in some people."

3. "Adverse Health Effects of Indoor Mold." *Journal of Nutrition and Environmental Medicine.* September 2004, 14(3), 271-274. Also see: Charlie Wiles, *Certified Microbial Consultant Review Course.* The American Indoor Air Quality Council, 2003, pp. 3, 8.

4. Sierck, Peter. *Mold Remediation in Nutshell.* Seminar sponsored by Environmental Microbiology Laboratory, June 2005. Also statements made by Chin Yang at *Current Understanding & Advancements in Mold Assessment, Sampling and Analysis.* Seminar. 2005.

    The author has not seen any data that bleach is effective in killing mold. The Clorox Company could not provide the author with the specifics of any testing performed in regards to any statements that bleach kills mold. When contacted, the Clorox Company responded, "We do apologize, we do not have the information you are looking for." [Clorox Company Reference Number: 4821634. February 2007].

    One study, funded by the Clorox Company, received a lot of attention after it was published: "Efficacy of sodium hypochlorite disinfectant on the viability and allergenic properties of household mold," *Journal of Allergy and Clinical Immunology:* Volume 113, Issue 2 (Supplement), Page S180 (February 2004). The abstract for this study does not state exactly how the study was performed and the full article is not available for purchase. John Banta of Restoration Consultants says that any reduction in the presence of mold may be due to cleaning (wiping the surface with a cloth and washing) vs. being neutralized by bleach.

The following study suggests bleach *is not* effective:

    "Our study results illustrate that the treatment [bleach] does not eliminate the surface micro flora [mold]," is the conclusion of the Oregon State University study of the effects of chlorine bleach on mold growth. (Professor Jeffrey Morrell. Department of Wood Science, Oregon State University. *Forest Products Journal:* 54:4, 2004).

    The ion structure of chlorine bleach may prevent it from penetrating into porous materials such as dry wall and wood. Sodium hypochlorite may stay on the surface of materials, whereas mold may have mycelium growing into the materials. Thus when you spray porous surfaces with bleach, the water in the solution soaks into it, while the chemicals stay on top. Considering this factor, even if bleach was effective in laboratory studies, any effectiveness might be limited to the surface layer and the water penetration into building materials may support further mold growth.

5. Grose, E., D. Costa, G. Hatch, R. Jaskot, and M. Stevens. "Chronic Exposure to Ozone Causes Restrictive Lung Disease." U.S. Environmental Protection Agency: Washington, D.C., EPA/600/D-89/102 (NTIS PB89224554) (cited online February 2007).

2 - PESTICIDES

WHAT IS IT?

By law, a pesticide is "any substance or mixture intended for preventing, destroying, repelling, or mitigating any pests." This includes insecticides, herbicides (weed killers), fungicides (mold killers), rodenticides, and antimicrobials.[1]

It is important to note what this definition does not include. Pesticides kill pests but they *do not* solve the pest problem. At best pesticides provide short-term respites from pests, and require repeated treatments to keep pest populations low.

Ingredients not on the Label

You may think you can determine how hazardous something is by reading the label. Forget about reading the label on a bottle of pesticides and making judgment calls. Typically there is only one or a few ingredients listed on the label. The rest are classified as "inerts." Almost 99% of the ingredients are typically labeled "inert." Inert does not mean harmless.

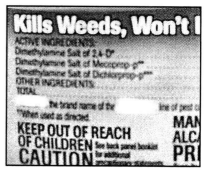

Typically only 1-2% of the total ingredients are listed on the label. Without knowing what's in them you can't make complete, informed decisions about health and safety.

Inert simply means an ingredient is not the primary chemical used to kill.

The manufacturer, not the EPA, decides what chemicals are inert. Many inert ingredients are more harmful than the active ones. Because many people have a misleading impression of the term *inert ingredient*, believing it to indicate

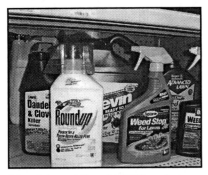

A few of the pesticide and herbicide products on the shelf at a local department store with the majority of the ingredients listed as inert or other ingredients. Inert and other do not mean harmless.

harmless ingredients, the EPA encourages manufacturers to substitute the more neutral term *other ingredients*.[2] By law, inert ingredients are considered trade secrets.

In a Freedom of Information Act lawsuit, the Northwest Coalition for Alternatives to Pesticides (NCAP) obtained from the EPA a list of 1,400 of the 2,000 substances currently being used as inert ingredients in pesticides. These included Chicago sludge, hazardous waste, asbestos, and some banned chemicals such as DDT.[3] Common inert ingredients include toluene, ethyl benzene, and xylene. These are central nervous system depressants and carcinogens.

WHAT CAN IT DO TO ME?

Pesticides have been reported as a leading cause of sinusitis, bronchitis, migraines, allergies, and immune system disorders such as chronic fatigue—even at low levels. Pesticides are known to cause birth defects, and there is a lot of evidence that suggests it causes breast cancer.

Children and pets are extremely vulnerable to pesticides. Children have more skin surface for their size than adults and have less mature immune and enzyme systems to detoxify chemicals.

The following picture demonstrates how pesticide exposure impairs neurological development in children exposed to pesticides.

The study compared drawings from children ages 4-5 that lived in an agricultural region where pesticides are applied. Most of their exposure came from pesticide drift and contaminated dust. The control group of children was from a nearby region and families that avoid the use of pesticides, using fly swatters to kill bugs.[4] The two groups are similar genetically, culturally, and physically.

In addition to impaired motor skills, another observation made in this study was that valley children (exposed) seemed less creative in their play. The valley children tended to roam the streets with minimal group interaction. Some valley children were observed hitting their siblings when they

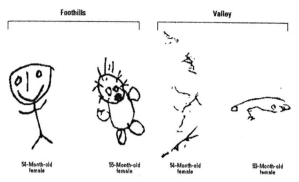

Drawings made by four-year-old children. The valley children (where pesticides are used) are not as neurologically developed as the foothills children where pesticides are not used. Reproduced with permission from Elizabeth A. Guillette and Environmental Health Perspectives.

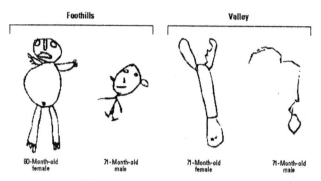

Drawings made by five-year-old children. The neurological development of the valley children (where pesticides are used) is impaired relative to the other children. Reproduced with permission from Elizabeth A. Guillette and Environmental Health Perspectives.

passed by and becoming easily upset or angry with minor corrective comments from parents. These aggressive behaviors were not noticed in the foothills children (unexposed).

There is a strong correlation between pesticides and cancer. Children in families that use pesticides are 6.5 times more likely to get childhood leukemia[5]. Pesticides are stored in fat tissues, build up, and can effect people years after exposure. Pesticide exposure has been associated with the following health problems:

- Immune system depressors [i.e. people get sick more often]

- Asthma and allergies

- Neurological disorders

- Learning disabilities

- Birth defects

- Breast cancer[6]

Of the thirty-four most commonly used lawn chemicals, eleven cause cancer, twenty cause nervous system poisoning, nine cause birth defects; and thirty cause skin irritation.[7] A component of Agent Orange, 2, 4-D, is used in about 1,500 lawn care products.[8] Roundup, a commonly used lawn-care product and weed killer is a pesticide. Despite claims that Roundup is safe, it is known to cause a variety of serious health problems.[9] Exposure to Glyphosate, the active ingredient in Roundup has been linked with an increased incidence of attention deficit disorder in children.[10] Most of the toxicity problems associated with Roundup, however, is not thought to stem from the active ingredient, Glyphosate, but from the unlabeled "inert" ingredients.

If you're a golfer it may be in your best interest to get your course to reduce their use of pesticides. Golfers are coming down with some unusual diseases in recent times. One study found mortality rates for golf course superintendents was high for four cancer types—brain, non-Hodgkin's lymphoma, prostate, and large intestine— a pattern similar to that found with workers in occupations exposed to pesticides.[11]

Mothballs contain dichlorobenzene, a carcinogen and a neurotoxin, that can harm the brain and cause depression. Mothballs are often responsible for health complaints during indoor environmental assessments.

WHERE IS IT?

The chemicals and solvents in pesticides can be detected long after application and long after sprays dry. If the chemicals applied didn't work after drying they wouldn't work to kill the weed or pest. You'd be calling the exterminator back the next day.

Potentially harmful chemicals are in the pesticides the exterminator applies, even in the newer, "safer" water-based pesticides. Because all of the ingredients are not listed on the label, even the exterminator does not know what is really in them.

Pesticides attach to dust. **Contrary to popular belief, the major pathway that pesticides get into your body is not from breathing vapors**

while spraying pesticides but through your skin from contact with contaminated dust.[12]

Using pesticides in the house or in the yard creates the potential for cumulative buildup over time. Studies have show that urban soils have higher levels of pesticides than agricultural areas.[13] Pesticides attach to the bottom of shoes and are tracked into the house. Since pets and children spend more time in contact with floors, carpets, and other dusty surfaces, they potentially have more exposure.

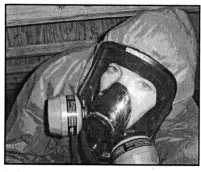

You've got to protect yourself. Not from spiders — from pesticides. Dust is the major pathway by which the body is exposed to pesticides. Pesticides can remain in the soil for 20 years or more.

Mothballs are horribly toxic. Mothballs are nearly 100 percent dichlorobenzene and naphthalene.[14] Upon breathing vapors from mothballs these chemicals quickly enter the bloodstream. If you are in a room with mothballs your clothing and skin will absorb the chemicals. Deodorizer blocks labeled as "cedar," "pine," or "lavender" may consist primarily of paradichlorobenzene. Being a derivative of the mothball chemical, it is also easily absorbed.

Furnace ducts leaks 30% on average. This means if there is ductwork in the crawlspace some portion of the air inside in a home may be contaminated with pesticides sprayed in the crawlspace.

While we think of pesticides as temporary solutions to various pest problems, they linger sight and scent unseen, both inside and outside.

GET RID OF IT!!!

Keep it simple: under most circumstances you should not need to use pesticides. What is the pest you are trying to kill? When was the last time you saw it? Don't just have the exterminator come once a month.

Twenty of twenty-five common pests are only a problem because their natural predators have been killed by pesticides.[15] If you have bugs, formulate a strategy to combat the bug for which you have the problem. Don't apply a blanket pesticide to kill everything.

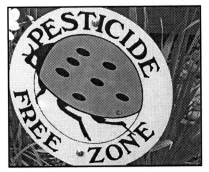

Be a trend setter. This Pesticide-Free Zone sign can be ordered from the Washington Toxics Coalition, (206) 632-1545, www.watoxics.org.

Identify why you have a bug problem. Ants and cockroaches are attracted to food and moisture. You may have a hidden plumbing leak somewhere.

Is the bug problem a threat to your health or just a nuisance? Spiders, except for the black widow and the brown recluse, do not pose a threat to humans. Chemicals are not effective in combating spiders. They will come back as long as conditions are attractive.

Start with the least toxic pest control method. This may be some sort of trap or bait. Sticky bait traps have pheromones to attract pests. Monitor the effectiveness of these and only proceed to something more toxic if other methods don't work.

If you need to use pesticides, try the least-toxic pesticide first. Look for a product for which all of the ingredients are listed on the label. If all of the ingredients are not listed, if there are any "inert" ingredients, do not use it.

Having an EPA registration does not make something safe. The EPA approves a pesticide based on it doing what it says it will do, not safety.[16] If a product is very effective the EPA will tolerate higher health and environmental risks and approve the product.

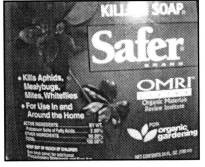

While this product may appear safer, 98% of the ingredients are listed as inerts. Do not buy anything unless ALL of the ingredients are listed on the label.

Least-toxic pesticide ingredients include:

- Boric acid to combat ants, termites, fleas, roaches (also a good mold-inhibitor)

- Diatomaceous earth to kill scorpions, crickets, and other insects

- Sticky traps for ants and moths.

Boric acid dries out and breaks down the exoskeleton of insects. It is good for flea control. Sprinkle on the carpet, not the dog.

Getting Rid of Ants

- Vacuum up the ants with a vacuum cleaner or wipe them up with a wet sponge.
- They get lost without a trail. Spray the scent trail with hydrogen peroxide. Follow the trail and pour boiling water into the nest (ouch!).
- Use bait traps. Boric acid is a less-toxic alternative to harsher chemicals. A home-made version can be made by mixing 1 teaspoon boric acid, 6 table-spoons granulated sugar and two cups of warm water. Place on a cotton ball and put in the bottom of a plastic cup with holes cut in for ants to enter. This is also good for roaches. Put it under the refrigerator. Keep out of reach of children and pets.

Lawn Care

Tips for a Healthier, Non-toxic Lawn

Healthier grass will resist pests on its own, without the use of pesticides. Don't give your lawn "junk food" in the form of commercial fertilizers. It stresses the lawn and makes it more vulnerable to pests.

- Use organic compost for fertilizer. Make your own compost pile with kitchen scraps. It's fun for the kids.

- Do not cut grass too short. Two to three inches is best.

- Do not over-water. Give your lawn slow, deep watering.

- Weed by hand—it's good exercise!

- Daises, sunflowers, marigolds, dill, and fennel attract beneficial insects like praying mantis and lady bugs which eat other bugs.

- Safer alternatives for controlling weeds are corn gluten, hot water, and vinegar, weed-whackers, and mowing.

Moths

Don't confuse the moths you see flying around near the light at night with clothes moths. Clothes moths are quite small, and when disturbed will run or fly to conceal themselves. Dry-cleaning is effective at killing. Running clothes through the dryer kills moths.

Storing clothes in airtight containers such as cedar chests or in bags sealed with tape is effective at keeping larvae out. It is important to clean your clothes before you store them. If clothes are packed with even one egg the moth larvae will survive.

Remember: pesticides kill pests but they do not solve the pest problem. There are many safe, creative means of controlling little creatures that infest or disturb your environment.

Fred's Bugs

I always wear a respirator and a moon-suit whenever I go into a crawlspace. Most people assume it's because of mold. It's actually because of pesticides.

Most crawlspaces have been sprayed with pesticides at one time or another. Some older types of pesticides can last thirty years before breaking down. Newer types of pesticides can last a long time, too. To "break" down simply means the chemicals in the formulation come unglued from each other. The original ingredients are still there, perhaps more harmful in their broken down state.

Such was the case at Fred's house. Fred and his wife contacted me to test for mold. Fred had a persistent rash that would not go away. Their home was a clean as a button. Sparsely furnished with hard wood floors, Wilma must have vacuumed twice a day because I had a hard time collecting a dust sample. I checked the home for water damage and took some air samples to test for mold. The tests indicated a very clean environment.

I asked Fred if he used pesticides. With enthusiasm Fred explained how determined he was to kill the bugs and what a constant battle it was. He routinely sprayed pesticides. He did this himself, with no protection. He mixed the pesticides in a large spray canister, and rather than diluting it per the instructions, he figured a higher strength would work better.

I suggested that since pesticides are known to cause skin rashes that he stop using them for a while and see if his rash went away. He did. It took several months but his rash subsided. His bug problem also went away. When I asked him, he couldn't remember what the bug problem was.

RESOURCES
Natural Gardening Guidebook
One of the best books currently available on the subject is *Natural Gardening: A Guide to Alternatives to Pesticides*, published by the state of Oregon and the City of Portland Metro (503) 234-3000. A copy can be down-loaded for free www.metro-region.org/garden

When you get to the website do a search on "natural gardening guidebook". This might seem like a lot of effort but it's worth it.

Propane torch kit to kill weeds
Hooks up to any propane tank (barbeque cylinders work great).
Flame Engineering, Inc.
Phone: (888) 388-6724
Web Site: http://www.flameengineering.com/Weed_Dragon.html
For details see: http://www.pesticide.org/pubs/alts/pdf/flameweeding.pdf

The Northwest Coalition for Alternatives to Pesticides (NCAP)
Maintains a large library of free, on-line fact sheets and a hot line for those who prefer to order them by mail order or get phone support regarding alternatives to pesticides. Support them by becoming a member.
Phone: (541) 344-5044
Website: pesticide.org
E-mail: info@pesticide.org

The Washington Toxics Coalition
Loads of helpful information including downloadable files "Talking to your Neighbors about Pesticides," and the Pesticide Free Zone sign to put in your yard.
Phone: (206) 632-1545
Website: www.watoxics.org
E-mail: info@watoxics.org

The Bio-Integrated Resource Center
Specializing in non-toxic and least-toxic, Integrated Pest Management (IPM) solutions. Free, on-line fact sheets. Training for professionals. Want to make your golf course non-toxic? These are the people to ask for help.
Phone: (510) 524-2567
Website: http://www.birc.org

Care2.com
Care2 is a large online resource that includes tips for non-toxic pest control.
Web site: http://www.care2.com/channels/lifestyle/home#52

SUGGESTED READING
The Healthy School Handbook, National Education Association (NEA) Professional Library publication, Washington, D.C., 1995.

Lynn Dadd, Debra, *Home Safe Home*, Penguin Putnam Inc., New York, 1997, p.108.

Moses, Marion, M.D., *Designer Poisons, How to Protect Your Health and Home from Toxic Pesticides*, Pesticide Education Center, San Francisco, CA, 1995.

END NOTES

1. "What is a Pesticide?" *Journal of Pesticide Reform*. Northwest Coalition for Alternatives to Pesticides, summer 1999, Vol. 19. No.2.
2. Environmental Protection Agency. *Pesticide Registration Notice 97-6*. http://www.epa.gov/opppmsd1/PR_ Notices/pr97-6.html (cited online July 2006).
3. Baker-Laporte, Paula, Erica Elliot, M.D., and John Banta. *Prescriptions for a Healthy House*, New Society Publishers, 2001, p. 10. For more information on the secret ingredients in pesticides see NCAP's website: Pesticde.org/factsheets.html#pesticides.
4. Guillette, Elizabeth A., et al. "An Anthropological Approach to the Evaluation of Preschool Children Exposed to Pesticides in Mexico." *Environmental Health Perspectives, the National Institute of Environmental Health Sciences*, V.106, N.6, June, 1998.
5. Children's Health Environmental Coalition. *The Household Detective Primer, Protecting you children from toxins in the home*. 2000, p.14.
6. A recent study published online in the American Journal of Epidemiology (December 2006), found a strong link between residential pesticide use and breast cancer risk in women. *Reported Residential Pesticide Use and Breast Cancer Risk on Long Island, New York*. http://aje.oxfordjournals.org/cgi/content/abstract/kwk046v1 (cited online January 2007).

The biggest risk factor for breast cancer is estrogens, female hormones. Pesticides mimic natural estrogens found in the body and disrupt hormone activity. Pesticides accumulate in fat tissue. Over time chronic exposure results in higher levels stored in the body. (Moses, Marion, M.D. *Designer Poisons, How to Protect Your Health and Home from Toxic Pesticides*. Pesticide Education Center, San Francisco, CA, 1995, p.79).

Other sources for the statement that pesticides contribute to breast cancer include:

Pesticides and Breast Cancer. April, 1996. National Coalition for Alternative to Pesticides (NCAP). http://www.pesticide.org/BCancerReport.pdf.

"Pesticide Residuals and Breast Cancer: The Harvest of a Silent Spring?" *Journal of the National Cancer Institute*, April 21, 1993, pp. 598-599.

Guillette, Elizabeth A., et al. "Altered Breast Development in Young Girls from an Agricultural Environment." *Environmental Health Perspectives*, 114:471-475(2006).

7. Bong, Jennifer. "Children at risk – Widespread Chemical exposure Threatens Our Most Valuable Population." *E-Magazine*, September/October 2001, p. 36.
8. Baker-Laporte, *Prescriptions for a Healthy House*, p. 11.
9. Mendelson, Joseph. "Roundup: The World's Best-Selling Herbicide." *The Ecologist*, Volume 28 No 5, September/October 1998, p. 270.
10. Cox, Caroline, ed. "Herbicide Fact sheet, Glyphosate" and "Glyphosate, Part 1: Toxicology." *Journal of Pesticide Reform*, NCAP.
11. "Golf Course Superintendents Face Higher Cancer Rates." *American Journal of Industrial Medicine*, 29(5):501-506, 1996.
12. Moses, Marion, M.D. Designer Poisons, How to Protect Your Health and Home from Toxic Pesticides, p. 20.
13. Ibid., p 30.
14. Washington Toxics Coalition. Fact Sheet, "Clothing Moths – Prevention and Control." *Alternatives*. http://www.watoxics.org/files/clothingmoth.pdf (cited January 2007).
15. CHEC, The Household Detective Primer, Protecting you children from toxins in the home, p. 14.
16. Moses, Designer Poisons, p.19.

3 - FRAGRANCE

WHAT IS IT?

Fragrance is used to make things smell good. Historically fragrance was first used in religious rituals in which someone or something was *cleansed* from evil spirits or where offerings were made to a God. Thus began the association between something smelling clean and being good.

In modern times, this association persists, even though we know that something can be quite dirty when it smells clean. In fact, fragrance is used to mask odors from the garbage can, cat box, and bathroom.

Fragrance can be made using natural ingredients or essential oils, but more often it is made using synthetic chemicals. As many as 600 separate chemicals may be used in a single fragrance formula, the list of which is protected as a trade secret. According to the Food and Drug Administration, about 4,000 different chemicals are used in the fragrance industry. The most common ingredients in fragrance are toluene—detected in every sample collected by the EPA—formaldehyde, acetone, benzene, and methyl chloride.

Some of the chemicals in fragrance are odorless, *fixatives* that slow the evaporation rate of the fragrant compounds. These include diethyl phthalate—a toxic, eye, and mucus membrane irritant—

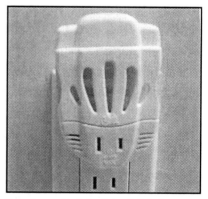

Drug therapy. The bulk of chemicals in fragrances are petro- chemicals similar to gasoline with a bit of "artificial fragrance" added. What does breathing gas fumes 24 hours a day do to you?

benzopherone, synthesized from benzene, and propylene glycol (antifreeze). Some of these same chemicals are used in the pesticide industry.

Fragrance is a poison. The replacement package for plug-in air fresheners reads "warning...if swallowed, call poison control."

WHAT CAN IT DO TO ME?

The chemicals in fragrance are neurotoxins and suppress the immune system. In one laboratory experiment mice were exposed to fragranced air, 5 out of 186 mice died.[1] A study by the National Institute of Occupational Safety and Health (NIOSH) found that in a particular list of 2,983 chemicals being used in the fragrance industry, 844 toxic substances were identified.

Chemicals in fragrance can trigger asthma and allergies and cause neurological, liver, and kidney damage. According to the FDA, fragrance causes 30% of all allergic reactions.[2] An estimated 50 million Americans or perhaps one in five, have some degree of health problem associated with fragrance exposure.[3] Scientists think that chemicals in fragrances may be endocrine disrupters, producing the same effects in the body as pesticides. Studies done with computer imaging have shown abnormal blood flow in the brain after exposure to perfume.[4]

WHERE IS IT?

Artificial fragrances are in household cleaners, laundry detergent, fabric softener, air fresheners, and personal care products. The biggest sources of exposure in the home are plug-in type air fresheners and laundry soap. At the office and school, personal perfume and cologne are big sources of exposure.

Plug-in type air fresheners contain naphthalene, phenol, cresol, ethanol, xylene, and formaldehyde. Some people have these chemicals spewing into the air in homes and offices twenty-four hours a day. The irony is that the chemicals in air fresheners diminish the ability to smell.[5]

Laundry soap contains a high level of fragrance. The makers of laundry soap think that *you* think your clothes have to smell good in order to be clean. When you wash with fragrant laundry soap, you end up breathing chemicals

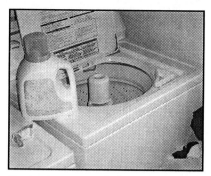
Most laundry soaps contain fragrance.

the whole time you are wearing your clothes and when you are sleeping in bed on bedding and sheets washed in fragrance. This adds up to you being exposed to the chemicals in fragrance a significant amount of your time.

Chemicals attach to fibers, especially synthetic ones. Every time clothes are washed more chemicals are added. It can be difficult to wash fragrance out once it gets into fabrics. People who have had their bedding for a long time can have a significant accumulation of chemicals in the fabric.

Some laundry soap is marketed specifically for babies. Unfortunately, unless other wise noted on the label, these too contain fragrance. One such brand is Dreft® which also advertises it does not rise out fire retardants. This may seem like a good thing unless you consider that flame retardants are toxic. Researchers are finding toxic health effects from flame retardants. Children are most at risk, receiving up to 300 times greater exposure than adults.[6] Legislation in the State of Washington is calling for a ban on toxic flame retardants. There are alternatives.

GET RID OF IT!!!

Keep it simple: you don't need fragrance in everything. The placebo effect from things smelling clean is not worth the physical harm chemicals in fragrance have on your body. For those places you do want fragrance, essential oils are a healthier alternative.

There is no way for a consumer to know which chemicals are in a fragrance. If you see the word *fragrance*, don't buy it.

Don't use synthetic air fresheners, especially plug-in type air fresheners.

Determine what the source of a bad odor is and eliminate it rather than mask it with a fragrance.

Make your own aerosol deodorant. Fill a spray bottle with water mixed with a few drops of your favorite essential oil (about 100 drops to 1 cup water). Essential oils can be found at health food stores and online. Organic, therapeutic grade essential oils are recommended for purity. Pick a scent that you like. To create a very potent mixture, use vinegar instead of water. Vinegar can burn the eyes. Keep this mixture out of reach of children.

Baking soda and borax absorb odors. Add a few drop of your favorite essential oil to a box of Arm & Hammer and place it near the cat box or mix with the litter. Sprinkle a 1/8-cup of the mixture in the bottom of the trash can.

The best thing you can do for your family is to **_stop washing cloths and bedding with fragrant laundry detergent_**. Buy _fragrance-free_ laundry soap. While it helps to read the label, you can't trust the label. Fragrance free does not mean no added fragrance. Fragrance can be added to neutralize the odor of the fatty acids used to make soap. There is no government definition for _fragrance-free_.

Your best options are to smell the soap and buy from companies that list all of the ingredients on the label with no added fragrance. These include Seventh Generation, Ecover, Earth's Best, Earthrite, Earth Friendly, Bio Kleen, Life Tree, and Dr. Bronner's Soap, to name a few.

Perfume and cologne affect everyone around those who wear it. If you need to wear a fragrance consider ones made with a blend of essential oils and use them sparingly. The Fragrane Foundation, supported by the fragrance industry has an "Arm's Length Rule." A person an amr's length away should not be able to realise you are wearing any.[7]

The Healthy School Handbook states that school attendance can improve, and academic achievement increase, if an effort is made to remove all perfumed products from the classroom setting.

Sniff-Sleuthing

Rob and Kathy had just moved out of a rental home where they had experienced mold problems. Their next home appeared to be dry and free of mold, but they were experiencing headaches and foggy thinking. Their familiarity with mold made them suspect mold again, and they called me to investigate.

I sniffed around and the only thing I found wrong was the carpet. The landlord had cleaned the carpet before they moved in, but I picked up traces of pet odors. The previous tenant probably had an indoor pet, and the carpet cleaning company probably had to work extra hard to eliminate the pet odors. I suggested they re-clean the carpet. Just rinsing it with water would help. If not, the carpet would need to be replaced.

I had a similar experience myself staying in a hotel room while on a business trip. I was staying up late, working at the desk in my room next to the bed. I kept smelling fragrance that I attributed to the cleaning staff. I figured it would go away if I opened a window. It was the middle of winter, so leaving the window open all night wasn't an option.

I aired out the room but still smelled the fragrance. It started to give me a headache and made it difficult to concentrate on my work. A big source of fragrance is pillows and sheets so I sniffed the bedding. It smelled fine except for a decorative throw blanket on the end of the bed. I put the blanket in the closet and went back to work.

Still no relief. Finally I smelled the carpet. It was highly fragrant. They had just washed the carpet. Perhaps, similar to Rob and Kathy's home, they had to use something fragrant to hide the odor. I had them move me to another room and there was no problem.

Rob, Kathy, and I are not chemically sensitive. The chemicals in fragrance affect everyone's nervous system. Sure, I could have survived a night in my original hotel room, but I choose not to do drugs. My sniff-sleuthing solved the problem.

RESOURCES

Essential oils
Young Living Essential Oils
Phone: (800) 371-3515
Web site: http://www.youngliving.us

Frontier/ Simply Organic/ Aura Cacia
Phone: (800) 669-3275
Web site: http://frontierherb.com/dspCatTxt.php?ct=anpceoeo

Zeolite
Zeolites are naturally occurring, volcanic ash minerals that are uniquely effective in the control of odors including ammonia from pets. Order from *Eco Clean*.
Phone: (866) 287-6892 or (480) 947-5286
Web site: http://www.ecoclean-az.com

SUGGESTED READING

Fragrance and Health, by Louise A Kosta. May be found on Amazon.com or ordered from the publisher, the Human Ecology and Action League (HEAL). Member price: $12.00; others $24.00. HEAL annual membership includes 4 issues of *The Human Ecologist.* US: $26.00 (low income $20.00); Canada $32.00.
Website: http://members.aol.com/HEALNatnl/index.html
Phone: (404) 248-1898.
Mail orders to:
HEAL
PO Box 29629
Atlanta GA 30359-1126

The Healthy School Handbook, Conquering the Sick Building Syndrome and Other Environmental *Hazards in and around Your School,* National Education Association (NEA) Professional Library publication, Washington, D.C., 1995.
Phone: (800) 229-4200. Stock No. 1866-4-00-C4

FOOT NOTES

1. Kosta, Louise A. *Fragrance and Health.* The Human Ecology Action League (HEAL), 1998, p. 46.
2. Miller, Norma L., Ed.D, ed. *The Healthy School Handbook.* National Education Association Professional Library publication, Washington, D.C., 1995, p. 70.
3. Fragrance and Health, pp. 34, 38.
4. The Healthy School Handbook, p. 71.
5. Ibid., p. 71.
6. "Bills to Eliminate Toxic Flame Retardants Off to A Fast Start." *Alternatives.* Washington Toxics Coalition, Seattle, WA, Winter 2007, Volume 26, No. 1.
7. Frasrance and Health p. II.

4 - CLEANING SUPPLIES

WHAT IS IT?

Chemicals in cleaning supplies include alcohol, ammonia, bleach, formalde-hyde, petroleum derivatives, phenols, glycols, chlorine, and fragrance.

Some companies will engage in "green washing," a practice where they make their product *appear* to be non-toxic. One example is Simple Green, which from its name to its advertising is marketed as a safe, non-toxic alternative cleaner. Yet it contains butyl cellosolve, a compound found in cleaners like Formula 409 and Windex.[1] You won't know this by reading the label.

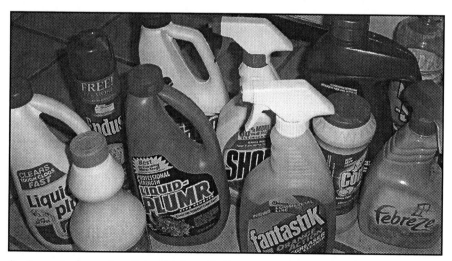

Cleaning supplies from under a kitchen sink in a typical household. How do you know which chemicals are in them? Very few if any ingredients are listed the label.

Another example is *Zen* general purpose cleaner found at Trader Joe's. This one lists alcohol on the label but because of the green packaging the average consumer is unlikely to read the label and might assume it does not contain any potentially harmful ingredients.

Cleaning products have been regulated by the Consumer Produts Safety Commission since the Federal Hazardous Substances Labeling Act in 1960. There are so many loopholes in this regulation that manufactures can often put a single, general warning on a label instead of listing specific toxic ingredients. Reading labels would be humorous if these products didn't have significant potential to seriously affect your health.

For example, the following ingredients were listed on a bottle of general purpose cleaner found at a chain grocer: "Ingredients: cleaning agents, quality control agents, perfume, colorant and water." Obviously quite vague.

WHAT CAN IT DO TO ME?

The chemicals in cleaning supplies are known to aggravate allergies and initiate asthma attacks. Within seconds of exposure, traces of these chemicals can be found in the body. The chemicals may irritate eyes, nose, and throat and cause headache, nausea, and neuro-toxic effects.[2]

A 15-year study found that women who work at home have a 54% higher rate of cancer than those who work away from home as a direct result of exposure to chemicals in common household products.[3]

WHERE IS IT?

Wherever cleaning supplies with hazardous chemicals are used, the air in the room is affected for hours afterwards.

GET RID OF IT!!!

Keep it simple. It's not necessary to have all these chemicals to clean effectively. Use plain soap and water or the least toxic cleaning supply that will get the job done.

Use as little cleaning product as possible. There are many surfaces for which a simple dusting with a damp cloth is sufficient and a cleaning agent is not necessary.

Don't bother with anti-microbial soaps and bleach. They don't work. Don't worry about germs. Bacteria are everywhere. Pathogenic bacteria and viruses are not normally present indoors. Claims about disinfectants and anti-microbial products killing germs are questionable. The EPA does not test disinfectants before registering them. The government found 20% of disinfectant products do not work.[4]

Read the label but don't make decisions based solely on reading the label. Reading the label on a cleaning product is similar to reading one on a bottle of pesticides: there may be one or two *active* ingredients. The rest are called *inert* or *other* ingredients. Inert does not mean safe.

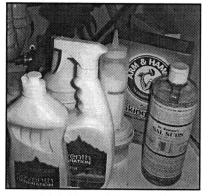

There are no government regulations on what can be labeled safe, natural, or green. Be wary of the words *safe, natural, non-toxic,* and *bio-degradable.* These are not regulated terms. Bio-degradable can mean hundreds of years.

There are many brands of non-toxic cleaning supplies that list *all* of the ingre-

Cleaning supplies from under the kitchen sink in a healthier home. All you need to clean: basic soap, vinegar, and borax. All of the ingredients are listed on the labels.

dients on their labels. These include: Seventh Generation, Ecover, Earth's Best, Earthrite, Earth Friendly, Bio-Kleen, Life Tree, and Dr. Bronner's Soap to name a few. They can be found at local health food stores as well as many chain grocery stores.

Choosing at the Grocery

- If you see the words *Warning, Hazardous, Caution,* or *Harmful*—stop! That's an indication that there is a safer product to be found.

- Don't buy it unless ALL of the ingredients are listed.

- Avoid what appear to be synthetic ingredients such as chlorine and benzene. These are identified on the label beginning with *chlor* or ending with *ene*.

- Avoid products with anti-microbials. This is a sign that the product contains chemicals not listed on the label.

- Ask your parents what they used. The old-fashioned way of cleaning worked and was typically less toxic than today's.

- Trust you nose and use common sense.

Homemade Cleaners and Disinfectants

Vinegar removes dirt and cuts grease. Excellent to clean windows with. An effective floor cleaner can be made by mixing liquid soap with one-quarter cup of vinegar to a gallon of water.

Vinegar is one of the most powerful anti-microbials on the planet and effectively kills bacteria and viruses. Make a mixture in a plastic spray bottle consisting of a few tablespoons of vinegar to a few cups of water. Use it to spray cutting boards and surfaces in the kitchen.

Baking soda is a natural deodorizer. Add a few drops of your favorite essential oil, sprinkle on carpets and vacuum up. Baking soda, mixed with hot water, is good for scrubbing and it deodorizes.

Lemon juice helps remove grease and sludge.

Borax has effective mold inhibiting properties. Mix 1 cup borax to a gallon of hot water for general cleaning. A paste of it can be applied to wood to aid in preventing mold, rot, and termites.

Borax can be added to the laundry to disinfect mold and odors. Borax boosts the cleaning power of normal detergents. It helps with hard water by breaking down the minerals that interfere with the cleaning agents in the detergent.

Borax is one of the ingredients in a popular laundry detergent marketed specifically for babies (unfortunately this product also contains fragrance and other chemicals). Make your own baby detergent. Pre-soak and pre-wash new baby cloths by adding ½ cup borax to a non-toxic laundry soap.

A mixture of olive oil and beeswax makes a good furniture polish. Clean the dust off the furniture first using a damp cloth then apply the oil and wax mixture to protect the wood.

RESOURCES

Your body is your best resource to help you determine how safe a product is for you. The following is a simple way to test your body's reaction to a product:

1. Hold either arm straight out from your side.

2. Have a partner place their hand on your arm just above your wrist. Now hold your arm firm as your partner gently pushes down. Do not use excessive force to resist. Notice how much pressure it takes your partner to push your arm down.

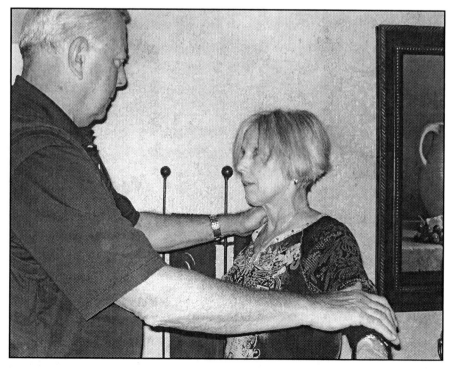

Using your body to evaluate if you are sensitive to something

3. Now relax your arm.

4. Have your partner place in your *other* hand the product to be tested. This arm can hang loose by your side while holding the product or thing to be tested.

5. Hold your free arm out again, firm. Have your partner gently push down again. If your arm goes weak, your body is having a negative reaction to something in the product.

This test method is called *Applied Kinesiology*. When a substance comes in contact with a person who is allergic to it, its properties will block the body's flow of energy resulting in weakened muscles. For a very interesting experience, try this with your cell phone as the product being tested.

From War to Wash

How many of you have had the unpleasant experience of breathing chlorine fumes while cleaning with bleach? We generally hold our breath thinking it's got to be done because the benefit of killing the germs is worth the cost of breathing the fumes. But is it necessary? When did we start thinking it was necessary to put up with the smell of chemicals to have a clean and "safe" home?

Chlorine gas is highly unstable and was difficult to produce until around World War I. While trying to manufacture chlorine gas for chemical weapons, it was found that breaking down salt water using electricity produced a compound called sodium hypochlorite - *bleach*.

The German army first used chlorine gas in 1915 against the French at Ypres. Chlorine gas destroyed the respiratory organs of its victims and led to a slow and horrible death by asphyxiation. After the first attacks, allied troops were supplied with masks of cotton pads that had been soaked in urine. It was found that the ammonia in the pad neutralized the chlorine.[6]

America's first commercial-scale liquid bleach factory was founded in the San Francisco Bay area. The plan was to convert the brine in salt ponds into bleach. It required massive amounts of electricity. As in modern times, the manufactures were able to buy electric power at cheap prices to make it profitable to produce chlorine bleach.

At first the product was not a success and retailers were instructed to hand out three of every four bottles free.[7] Thanks to extensive national advertising, bleach became commonplace.

Chlorine is very toxic and is a common link in many of the most notorious poisons: dioxin, DDT, Agent Orange, and ozone-depleting CFCs.

There are many alternatives to chlorine. For whitening clothes there is oxygen bleach (peroxides). For drinking water there is ultraviolet light, ozone, copper and silver ionization, and improved filters. Many large cities in Europe and Los Angeles, California use these to supplement or replace the use of chlorine.

It's time to phase out the use of chlorine.

SUGGESTED READING

Berthold-Bond, Annie, *Clean and Green: The Complete Guide to Nontoxic and Environmentally Safe Housekeeping*, Ceres Press, 1994. Contains over 500 recipes for natural, homemade cleaning products.

Hollender, Jeffrey, *Naturally Clean; The Seventh Generation Guide to Safe & Healthy Non-toxic Cleaning*, New Society Press, 2005. A comparative list of the ingredients in conventional and non-toxic cleaning products.

Logan, Karen, *Clean House, Clean Planet – Clean your House for Pennies a Day, the Safe, Nontoxic Way*, Simon & Shuster, 1997.

Lynn Dadd, Debra, *Home Safe Home, Protecting Yourself and Your Family from Everyday Toxics and Harmful Household Products*, Penguin Putnam Inc., New York, 1997.

END NOTES

1. Hollender, Jeffrey. *Naturally Clean, The Seventh Generation Guide to Safe & Healthy, Non-Toxic Cleaning*. New Society Publishers, Gabriola Island, Canada, 2005, p. 71.
2. Children's Health Environmental Coalition, The Household Detective Primer, Protecting you children from toxins in the home, 2000.
3. Toronto Indoor Air Conference, 1990.
4. Miller, Norma L., Ed.D, ed. *The Healthy School Handbook*, p. 141.
5. Kail, Konrad, M.D. *Allergy Free, An Alternative Medicine Definitive Guide*. Alternative Medicine.com, Tiburon, California, 2000, p. 80.
6. *Chlorine*. http://www.spartacus.schoolnet.co.uk/FWWchlorine.htm (cited online February 2007).
7. The Clorox Company. *Company History*, http://www.thecloroxcompany.com/company/history/history2.html (cited online February 23, 2007).

5 - REMODELING

WHAT IS IT?

Chemicals are directly related to the rising surge of allergies around the world.[1] In the 1950s it was estimated that about 14% of the population suffered from allergies; today that estimate is between 40% and 75%. Why the dramatic increase? Allergists in Japan have proposed that chemicals act as sensitizing agents.

To test their hypothesis, they subjected two groups of mice to high levels of Japan's equivalent of juniper pollen. In both groups of mice, about 5% of the mice developed allergies to the pollen. They then exposed one of the groups to benzene from car exhaust fumes. Upon retesting the two groups of mice, the mice exposed to the car fumes showed a significant increase in allergic response to the pollen compared to the group not exposed to the car fumes.[2]

Remodeling can introduce lots of chemicals into the air. Here we will consider some of the top contenders affecting your health: paint, carpet, and kitchen cabinets.

A John Hopkins University study found that more than 300 toxic chemicals and 150 carcinogens are present in paint.[3] They include acetone, ammonia, benzene, formaldehyde, lead, pentachlorophenol, and xylene. Fresh paint will continue to emit chemicals like ethylene glycol for as long as three and one-half years.[4]

Carpet can have hundreds of different chemicals including formaldehyde, 4-phenylcylohexene, styrene, toluene, benzene, xylene, pesticides, and anti-fungicides.

Formaldehyde is in the glue that holds the different color scraps of carpet padding foam together. There is more formaldehyde in carpet padding than in the carpet itself. Rubber carpet backing contains vinyl and styrene-butadiene.

One of the biggest sources of the chemical pollution indoors is new kitchen cabinets. It is amazing how much formaldehyde kitchen cabinets can emit. The release of most formaldehyde may be within six months to one year. But after about a 50% decline, cabinets continue to emit formaldehyde for an indefinite period. It may take as long as ten years to get to outdoor levels. It's evident when the formaldehyde is finally evaporated from particleboard in mobile homes—the floor falls apart as if it were rotten.

WHAT CAN IT DO TO ME?

A study has found the prevalence of asthma to be related to emissions from newly painted indoor surfaces.[5] Paint contains ingredients know to lower sperm counts and cause sterility[6]. You don't need to breathe paint fumes to be affected. The chemicals are absorbed through skin on contact.

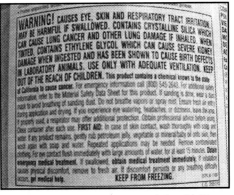
A typical can of paint. Does anyone read these labels?

According to Dr. Anderson of Anderson Laboratories, the chemicals emitted from carpeting can cause flu-like symptoms, fatigue, headaches, memory loss, and difficulty concentrating up to 16 weeks after exposure.[7] Dr. Anderson's laboratory exposes mice to samples of carpet to test carpet for toxicity.

Formaldehyde from kitchen cabinets can cause headache, fatigue, depression, asthma, and induce asthma attacks.[8] As many as 10% to 20% of people may be susceptible to formaldehyde at low concentrations.[9] Just because you don't smell anything doesn't mean these chemicals are gone. Most people get used to the way their home smells and the mind subsequently is programmed to ignore the smells.

GET RID OF IT!!!

Paint

Use zero-VOC paint. Most major brands carry a line of Zero-VOC paint. Paint can be low odor and still have high chemical content. There can be formaldehyde and acetone in low VOC paint. Ask the store for an MSDS (Material Safety Data Sheet). It won't list all the ingredients but it's a starting point. Call the paint manufacture and ask for full disclosure of all the ingredients.

If you really want to be healthy and creative try milk paint or a natural paint. You buy the pigment powders separately and mix them to create beautiful and unique colors. Milk paint is made from the casein protein of cows and does not contain petrol-chemicals.

Selecting a Paint

**Low & Zero VOC,
Trade Brands***
Benjamin Moore, *Pristine* Eco Spec
Sherwin Williams, *Health* Spec
Kelly-More, *Enviro-Cote*
Frazee, *Envirokote*
Glidden, *Lifemaster 2000*

**Low & Zero VOC,
Alternative Brands**
Chem Safe, (866)-287-6892, ecoclean-az.com
AFM, Safe Coat, (619) 239-0321, A popular line with the chemically sensitive.

Natural Paints**
Bio Shield, (800) 621-2591, BioShieldPaint.com
AGLAIA , (800) 322-6843, aglaiapaint.com
Auro Natural Paints, (888) 302-9352, Aurousa.com

Milk Paint
Old-Fashioned Milk Paint Company, (978) 448-6336, Milkpaint.com
BioShield, (800) 621-2591, BioShieldPaint.com
Real Milk Paint, (800) 339-9748, RealMilkPaint.com

*Low & Zero VOC Trade Brands - Some of these have ethylene glycol. Ask for a Material Safety Data Sheet.

**Natural Paints These brands make Zero VOC and natural paints. Some natural paints contain turpenes and citrus oils that smell and cause reactions in sensitive people.

Paint when the building is vacated and when you won't be home while it's drying. Open the windows during and after painting. ***Trust your nose***.

Carpeting

It is best to avoid carpeting. Consider hard wood flooring, tile, or manolium, a natural version of linoleum, instead. This improves air quality in other ways. Hard surfaces don't trap dust like carpets and are easier to clean.

Chose a carpet padding that does not contain formaldehyde. Jute and felt currently seem to be the only alternatives.

100% wool or other natural fiber, organic carpet is best. Lying on non-treated, wool carpeting (without insecticides, anti-microbials, moth-proofing, or stain treatments) is a treat.

Trust your nose. Choose the carpet with the least odor. If the sample in the store smells even a little, it's not a good choice. Bring it home and lay it in the sun for a few hours and smell it.

Look for carpet tested by Anderson Laboratories (ASTM E 981). This lab uses mice to test the health effects of being exposed to a carpet. www.andersonlaboratories.com/ (802) 295-7344.

Roll carpeting and padding out in the sun to air out prior to installing it. In office buildings, use low-VOC, *green* carpet glue.

If you have new carpet that stinks and you can't remove it, try applying AMF Carpet Guard.

Kitchen Cabinets

Particleboard is the worst offender. Choose cabinets made from solid wood, metal, or at minimum, exterior grade plywood.

If you don't have solid wood cabinets, seal the wood with Hard Seal, a sealant made by AFM. This requires two coats and getting all the nooks and crannies to be effective, something that can be very difficult to do once the cabinets are built.

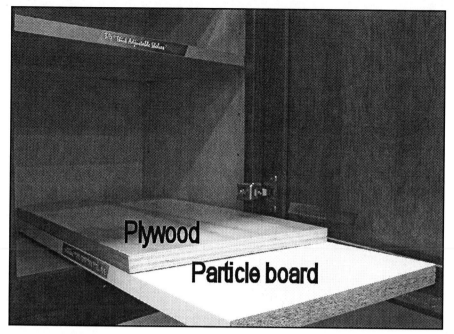

Often cabinets will have solid wood doors but the interior including the shelves are made with either plywood or particle board. Solid wood is preferred throughout. Plywood emits some formaldehyde; particle board emits a lot. By looking at the edge of the shelf you can distinguish plywood from particle board. Plywood has layers; particle board looks ground up.

New House Smell

New house smell it can be very difficult to get rid of without removing the sources (new carpet, cabinets, etc.)

Some people have tried to *bake-out* the house or use ozone or air purifiers to eliminate the odors. None of these may be effective.[10] Bake-outs involves heating the inside to at least 95°F for 48 hours and ventilating (opening the windows) afterwards. Bake-outs have little effect of reducing formaldehyde because of the thickness of materials. Bake-outs and ozone may damage materials, create new pollutants and odors, and cause condensation.

Air filters are of limited effectiveness. HEPA filters don't remove odors. Charcoal filters can't keep up with the rate that chemicals are being released from the materials.

You best bet is to remove the offending materials and build new homes with healthier materials and finishes.

The EPA Contaminates its Own

Carpet was in the media spotlight in 1988 when 125 employees at the EPA headquarters became ill after new carpet was installed. The chemical 4-PC, found in the latex backing, was thought to be responsible. The EPA replaced the carpeting with carpet that did not contain 4-PC but some employees continued to experience health problems. As a result, in 1992 the Carpet and Rug Institute, a trade association that represents about 95% of the carpet industry, formed the Green-Tag Program.[11]

When the Green-Tag program was created, it was criticized because it does not test for all of the toxic chemicals in carpet. Also only one sample from an entire product line was tested *once* per year. Several state attorneys general investigated and reported that there are insufficient testing standards to make safety claims about carpets.

In 2004, the program was modified. The Green Label Plus, as it is now called, includes testing for thirteen chemicals but does not ban the use of the chemicals.[12] Formaldehyde, Benzene, Styrene, and 4-PC are still allowed to be present in carpeting in amounts that may cause health problems.[13]

Tight but Toxic

While in transition from my job in construction to environmental consultant, I took a class at the community college where we helped build a house for Habitat for Humanity. The school was probably one of the best in the country for *green building*. Green building means saving the planet from impending doom by building as energy-efficiently as possible. This means making structure as airtight as possible to save on heating bills.

There is also some focus in *green building* on indoor air quality by choosing healthy paint, floor coverings, and other finishing. But while we could easily choose a low VOC paint, we had less budget and creative power to change the flooring materials or purchase different cabinets. At that time, we had even less experience understanding the significance of our choices.

We were on a tight schedule to finish building the house. In this case, the paint, vinyl flooring, budget-grade carpeting, and kitchen cabinets were all installed within a few days of each other. Even the workers who thought they weren't sensitive to chemicals were overwhelmed by the smell. And the house was air-tight!

The people that were fortunate enough to buy the home did not complain. They were just happy to own a home and probably not very knowledgeable about air quality either. Some people even like *new house smell*.

But what about the kids with allergies—kids on medication because allergies don't go away. Isn't it worth spending a little extra money for their health?

We couldn't afford healthy carpet but we could have had finished concrete floors instead of carpet and put shelves in the kitchen without doors instead of cabinets. This might sound stylistically bland, but some very high-end homes have been beautifully finished using these concepts.

RESOURCES

The *National Green Pages*™
An annual directory listing nearly 3,000 businesses. Free with membership.
Phone: (800) 58-GREEN. Search on-line by category and location at their web site:
http://www.coopamerica.org/pubs/greenpages.

The Architectural Resource Guide, edited by David Kibbey
An education directory of alternative building materials and suppliers. Order from the *Northern California Chapter of Architects, Designers and Planners for Social Responsibility.* P. O. Box 9126, Berkeley, CA 94709.
Phone: (510) 845-1000
Email: admin@adpsr-norcal.org
Website: www.adpsr-norcal.org

The Environmental Home Center
4121 1st Avenue South, Seattle, WA. If you're in the area, stop by their showroom. Otherwise browse online. Web Site: http://www.environmentalhomecenter.com
Phone: (206) 682-7332 or (800) 281-9785.

Eco Clean, The Healthy Home Solution
Natural carpet, non-toxic paint, AFM and other products for a healthier home.
2828 North 36th Street, Phoenix, Arizona
Web site: http://ecoclean-az.com
Phone: (480) 947-5286 or Toll-free (866) 287-6892.

AFM (American Formulating & Manufacturing)
Web site: www.afmsafecoat.com
Phone: (619) 239-0321.

SUGGESTED READING

Baker-Laporte, Paula, Erica Elliot, M.D., and John Banta, *Prescriptions for a Healthy House*, New Society Publishers, 2001.

Johnston, David, and Kim Master, Green Remodeling, Changing the World One Room at a Time, New Society Publishers, 2004.

END NOTES

1. Kail, Konrad, N.D., and Bobbi Lawrence. *Allergy Free, An Alternative Medicine Definitive Guide.* AlterntiveMedicine.com, Tiburon, CA, 2000, pp. 128-129. "According to Walter J. Crinnion, N.D., a researcher on environmental medicine, runaway chemical technology is directly related to the rising surge of allergies around the world. Before 1960 asthma was virtually non-existent in sub-Saharan African countries; today having turned to chemicals for agriculture and industry these countries have asthma rates equal to industrial countries."

2. Baker-Laporte, Elliot, and John Banta. *Prescriptions for a Healthy House.* New Society Press, 2001, p. 18. "Case Study 6: The experiment is described in "Adjutant activity of diesel exhaust particulates for the production of IgE antibody in mice" in the *Journal of Allergy and Clinical Immunology,* Vol. 77, April 1986, pp. 616-623.

3. Dadd, Debra Lynn. *Home Safe Home.* Penguin Putnam Inc, 1997, p. 312.

4. The Environmental Protection Agency Development of a Standard Test Method for VOC Emissions from Interior Latex and Alkyd Paints, EPA 600/R-01-093, November 2001, p. 128. http://www.epa.gov/appcdwww/iemb/EPA-600-R-01-093.pdf (cited online March 2007).

5. Wieslander, G., D. Norbaeck, E. Bjoernsson, C. Janson, and G. Boman. "Asthma and the indoor environment: The significance of emission of formaldehyde and volatile organic compounds from newly painted indoor surfaces." *International Archives of Occupational and Environmental Health,* vol. 69, no. 2, pp. 115-124, Jan 1997. http://pvc.buildinggreen.com/source.php?id=2268&sort=sourceName (Abstract cited online March 2007). Also see: EPA 600/R-01-093, p. 10.

6. Bower, John. *The Healthy House,* p. 391. References a 1991 issue of the *American Journal of Industrial Medicine* that found painters exposed to ethylene glycol in water-based paint had lower sperm counts.

7. Kail, Konrad, N.D., and Bobbi Lawrence. *Allergy Free, An Alternative Medicine Definitive Guide,* p. 136.

8. Godish, Thad, Ph.D. Director Indoor Air Quality Research Laboratory Indoor Air Quality Notes. *Formaldehyde – Our Homes and Health,* No. 1, 2nd Ed., Summer 1989. http://www.snowcrest.net/lassen/eiform1.html (cited online February 2007).

9. Bower, John. *The Healthy House,* The Healthy House Institute, Bloomington, IN, 1997, p. 39.

10. Ibid., pp. 186, 536.

11. Miller, Norma L., Ed.D, ed. *The Healthy School Handbook.* NEA (National Education Association) Professional Library publication, Washington, D.C., 1995, p. 183.

12. The Carpet and Rug Institute. *Green Label Plus – Carpet Testing Program.* http://www.carpet-rug.org/drill_down_2.cfm?page=8&sub=5&requesttimeout=350 (cited online July 2006).

13. California Department of Health Services. *Acceptable Emissions Testing for Carpet, Standard and Practice for the Testing of Volatile Organic Emission from Various sources Using Small-Scale Environmental Chambers.* California Department of Health Services, Indoor Air quality Section, California Specification 01350, July, 15, 2004, p. 55.

6 - DUST

WHAT IS IT?

Dust is more than dirt. About eighty percent of house dust is skin cells from people. A family of four produce about one quart of skin cells each month. Dust mites live off skin cells. Some people are allergic to the fecal matter dust mites produce.

Dust is also a complex mixture that contains particles from carpet, paint chips, cement and dust left over from construction and remodeling, pet allergens, cockroaches and mice feces, soot and tobacco smoke, mold spores, asbestos and fiberglass, lead, pesticides, weed and tree pollens, and dust carried in from miles away.

WHAT CAN IT DO TO ME?

If there is prevalence of something one is allergic to in the dust, these symptoms will be aggravated whenever the dust in a room is disturbed. If things are really dusty this can happen with a simple activity such as walking across the room or plopping down in a chair with fabric.

The most significant way dust is disturbed is by vacuuming and cleaning. Small particles can stay suspended for hours to days after vacuuming. Many of those with allergies or asthma have their symptoms triggered by vacuuming.

Even if you are not allergic to something in the dust, there is still potential harm a high level of small particles in the air caused by activities that stir up the dust. Small particles travel beyond the lungs and bloodstream, penetrating deep inside cells where they cause damage and disease.[1] This is thought to be what triggers asthma and heart attacks on hazy days.

WHERE IS IT?

Carpeting, upholstered furniture, blinds, bedding, and clutter hold dust. The dust that you can see is not as much as a health hazard as the small particles that are invisible. There may be hundreds of thousands of unseen particles in the air.

A common problem is dirty air filters. It is very common to find filters that have never been changed or are moldy. Commercial buildings may have a maintenance staff that takes care of this. But often when you ask, "Who takes care of changing the filters?" the reply is "We don't call someone unless there is a problem."

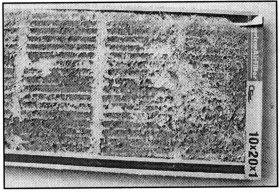

A dirty furnace air filter. No one knew where the filter was located so it never got changed. This is not uncommon in commercial buildings and even in residences.

GET RID OF IT!!!

Regardless of what the irritants and allergens in the dust may be, the remediation strategy is the same—a good old-fashioned cleaning, floor to ceiling. The trick is to minimize aerosolizing dust while you are cleaning.

Take the rugs, draperies, bedding, and pillows outside and beat them with a stick. This cleans much better than vacuuming. Throw the pillows in the dryer on fluff.

Vacuum the house thoroughly using a HEPA vacuum. A good vacuum cleaner is very important. If you don't have a good vacuum cleaner the level of fine particles in the air will increase when you're vacuuming causing more harm than good.

Damp wipe surfaces and mop with a damp cloth to both capture the dust and minimize aerosolizing fine particles.

Open the windows while dusting and vacuuming. If you have an air-purifier, turn it on during dusting and vacuuming.

Dust mites cannot live on food (skin cells) alone. They need moisture. Keep humidity below 50%.

Change the furnace air filter and upgrade it to an allergy-reduction type from 3M. Filters should be changed a minimum of every two months and more frequently if they look dirty when they are changed. Make sure the filter fits properly and that air cannot go around it.

Reducing the Need for Cleaning

- Take shoes off at the front door. Use a doormat.

- Furnish floors with wood, tile, or hard surfaces. Use rugs. Rugs are easier to wash than carpet on a regular basis.

- Get rid of clutter. Clutter collects dust, especially fabrics, fleecy materials, and papers.

- Minimize using the wood fireplace. Burning wood generates extremely high levels of dust particles. Wood smoke is more toxic than tobacco smoke.

Should You Get Your Ducts Cleaned?

Many people think that cleaning ducts will reduce dust. In fact, while dirty ducts can cause health problems, cleaning them may not lower dust levels indoors. This is because much of the dirt adheres to the surface of the ducts and does not enter the living space. You *should* consider having the ducts cleaned if they have never been cleaned and if they look dirty.

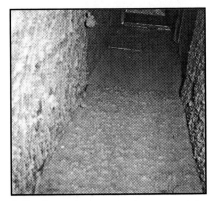

A dirty furnace duct.

When choosing a duct cleaning company make sure it is certified by the National Air Duct Cleaners Association (NADCA). A chemical sanitizer is not necessary. If things are effectively cleaned, there should be nothing left to sanitize. Especially avoid the use of fragrant or anti-microbial chemical sanitizers.

Lowering the amount of dust indoors is best accomplished by installing a good HEPA filter onto the furnace (see the chapter on air filters). This does not mean you won't have to dust anymore but possibly not as often. The reason you will still have to dust is that HEPA filters remove the very small particles. The larger particles settle out of the air quickly and show up as house dust. Remember, it's the small particles that have the most potential to affect your health.

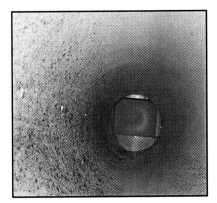

Mold inside a furnace duct. Courtesy: Martine Davis, Environmental Testing Inc.

Old Ducts, Old Dust

Kristy complained about mold to her landlord. She was renting part of a home that was very old. She thought the furnace and ductwork might have mold. There were ducts in the attic and supply vents on the ceiling to the bedroom and living rooms. She didn't have any problems until she turned the heat on at the beginning of winter. When she didn't run the heat there wasn't a problem.

Her landlord paid to have some testing for mold. The house was very old, and if you looked hard enough I'm sure you could eventually find some mold somewhere. But the results of air samples did not indicate any increase in mold indoors relative to the outside samples.

The landlord had the ducts cleaned and the complaints went away. The tenant was able to turn the heat on without having a reaction. This may not be too surprising considering the house was very old and the ducts had never been cleaned.

SUGGESTED READING
Kail, Konrad, N.D., and Bobbi Lawrence, *Allergy Free; An Alternative Medicine Definitive Guide*, www.AlterntiveMedicine.com, Tiburon, CA, 2000.

RESOURCES
Healthy Living Spaces
Visit the website: HealthyLivingSpaces.com
Call: toll-free (877) 992-9904, (505) 992-9904
HEPA Air Purifiers & vacuum cleaners

Vacuum Cleaners
Miele. Phone: (800) 843-7231 Website: www.miele.com
Nilfisk. Phone: (610) 647 6420 Website: http://nilfisk.com

Room Air Purifiers
The Health Pro Plus by IQ Air. Phone: (800) 500-4247. Website: www.IQAir.us

E.L. Foust Co., *Series 400* room air purifier and the *160AN* mobile unit for the car. Phone: (630) 834-4952. Website: www.foustco.com.

To find a certified duct cleaning company:
National Air Duct Cleaners Association (NADCA)
Phone: (202) 737-2926
Website: www.nadca.com
Email: info@nadca.com

END NOTES
1. Polakovic, Gary. *Air Particles Linked to Cell Damage.* Times Staff Writer, April 7, 2003, p. B7. Also http://www.iqair.us/research_air_particles_cell_damage.html (cited online July 2006).

See also: Shprentz, D.S. "Breath-Taking-Premature mortality due to particulate air pollution in 239 American cities." *Report of the Natural Resources Defense Council*, New York, NY, 1996.

7 - GAS

WHAT IS IT?

Natural gas or propane, as it is delivered to your home, contains many toxic ingredients. Gas comes from the ground. Like unfiltered tap water, it has impurities from the ground and from the gas supply lines. Some natural gas deposits have high concentrations of heavy metals, including lead, mercury, and arsenic. These accumulate on stove burners as black and white deposits.

There is a network of gas supply lines distributed across the country shared by different gas companies. You literally don't know where the gas supplied to your home comes from or what might be in it. Chemicals are either intentionally added or picked up including PCBs, dioxins, tars, oils, waxes, and plug-flow type chemicals. When these are burned, toxic stuff goes in the air. This is sporadic and appears in the flame as different colors.

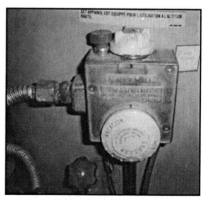

Many pilot controllers on gas hot water heaters leak, even when brand new. Get a warranty. It often cost more to repair them than replace the entire hot water heater.

When you burn natural gas, chemicals are created. Like an automobile engine, no gas appliance burns with 100% efficiency. Who likes to breathe exhaust from the tail pipe of a car? There is a long list of harmful chemicals with difficult-to-pronounce names produced when gas is burned. The biggest pollutants are carbon monoxide and formaldehyde.

WHAT CAN IT DO TO ME?

Natural gas has been found to be one of the most important sources of indoor air pollution. Natural gas can induce or worsen allergy, asthma, and chemical sensitivity.

Breathing even small amounts of gas compromises the immune system and increases the risk for asthma attacks, waking with shortness of breath, and tingling sensations in the extremities.

Lower concentrations of carbon monoxide may cause headaches, dizziness, nausea, and fatigue in healthy people. It causes chest pain in people with heart disease. At high concentrations it can cause unconsciousness and result in death.

If you don't smell gas you may think there's nothing to worry about. That is a bad assumption. Pure natural gas doesn't have an odor. Often there are chemicals from natural gas in the air at levels below what you can smell.

Water vapor is the produced when gas is burned. Chemicals attach to the water vapor. When you breathe the water vapor the chemicals are transported into your body.

WHERE IS IT?

In a study of 47,000 sensitive patients, the most important sources responsible for generating illness were the gas stove, the improperly vented gas water heater, and the gas furnace.[1]

There are practically no venting requirements for gas ranges, ovens, or clothes dryers. Gas ovens were installed with flues up until the 1950s. Now gas ovens and ranges are allowed to produce up to 800 ppm carbon monoxide without flues. There are no limits on the carbon monoxide emissions allowed from gas dryers or gas fireplaces.[2]

GET RID OF IT!!!

Make sure you gas appliances are venting properly and there are not leaks. If you smell gas there is a problem.

Your gas heater may have a heat exchanger that is corroded or cracked. This allows combustion gases to mix with the hot air supplied to the home instead of being exhausted outdoors. A home inspector can check this with a carbon monoxide probe.

Have a plumber test for gas leaks using a combustible gas meter. This is much more accurate than soap suds, the old-fashioned way. Pay particular attention to connections at pipe connections, the temperature controller on hot water heaters, and stove burners that do not shut off completely.

Open a window or turn on the exhaust hood when cooking with gas.

Replace Gas with Electric

The Canada Mortgage and Housing Corporation recommends replacing gas appliances with electrical appliances.[3] According to their studies, ventilating appliances did not seem to reduce health symptoms.

Debra Lynn Dadd, author of *Home Safe Home*, reports that many of her clients who do everything except remove gas from their homes have their symptoms from environmental sources remain. But almost as soon as they turn off gas appliances they start to feel better.[4] Dr. Alfred Zamm, author of *Why your House May Endanger your Health*, reports that a great many women have become sensitive to the fumes from gas stoves and when the gas range is replaced with an electric one, symptoms such as depression often disappear.[5]

The best thing to do is replace a gas water heater with an electric, on-demand,

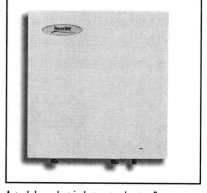

A tank-less, electric hot water heater. Pretty simple really. Takes up less space and has less potential for leaking and causing mold growth than conventional water heaters with storage tanks. Can be installed in a closet. Heats water instantly as needed. Photo courtesy: BBT North America, a Bosch Group company.

tank-less water heater. You can take a shower forever! They save money. Water is heated instantaneously and only when it is needed. Bosch is the brand that has been around a long time.

There are some other benefits to replacing gas with electric. You can install a timer on a standard electric hot water heater that will save you money by having it on only during times of peak usage. Using electric power may be more environmentally friendly than burning your own gas. Commercial power generating stations have technology that increases the energy efficiency of power generation.

If you have a wall-mounted gas heater, use portable, electric space heaters instead. The oil-filled ones that look like old radiant water heaters are very efficient. Because they radiate heat instead of heating the air they provide better comfort than gas heaters.

If you must have gas, properly ventilate. This means *sealed combustion* type units that include a fan to *power-exhaust* combustion air to the outdoors.

Maintain gas stoves.

The flame on stove burners should be blue. A persistent yellow-tipped flame means there is not enough oxygen, which means an increased amount of carbon monoxide and formaldehyde. A poorly adjusted gas stove can give off as much as thirty times more carbon monoxide and formaldehyde than a properly working one. Newer, pilot-less igniter type stoves are preferred to stoves with pilots that are continuously lit.

Install carbon monoxide detectors near gas furnaces and in hot water heater closets.

The Fallible Flex Hose

The furnace was located in the attic. To get to it I had to precariously climb a 20-foot ladder on the outside of the building. There, a small access panel allowed me to crawl into the attic. The homeowner, Alice, was sick and thought her house was killing her. My intention was to check for mold.

When I opened the panel to the attic I immediately smelled gas. It's a wonder that homes don't explode when they have gas leaks like this. I would have liked to shut the gas off, but the only way to tell where the leak was coming from was to leave it on, climb in, and investigate. They don't make a respirator that protects you against gas fumes so I tried to move quickly. I found that the flex hose that connected the gas supply pipe to the furnace was leaking.

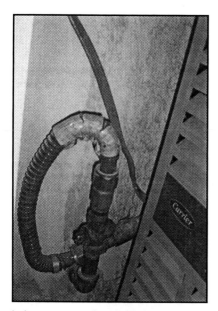

Leaks are common where flexible hoses connect the gas pipe line to appliances including furnaces, hot water heater, and stoves.

Alice called a plumber to fix it. The plumber replaced the hose. I asked him why not just tighten it. He replied that didn't always fix things and leaks can happen at any time, so better to start with a new hose. Considering this, you would think there would be a law requiring a gas detector capable of shutting the gas off in the event of a leak to be installed in places like this. No one goes into attics and crawlspaces on a regular basis just to check for gas leaks. Carbon monoxide detectors don't detect gas leaks.

At this time in my career I didn't know much about the health effects of natural gas and propane. I knew that breathing gas like I did in the attic was not good, but I didn't suspect it was be responsible for the home owner's health problems. So I was surprised when, later that night, she called me excited and explained how her research on the internet listed tingling in the extremities as a symptom of gas exposure. That was one of her prime health complaints with her doctor.

Propane is heavier than air and could have settled down into the home. More likely, the furnace was sucking air from the attic into the living space. Ductwork leaks. Furnace cabinets are not airtight.

SUGGESTED READING

Medical-Environment Report – A Review of the Potential Health Effects of the Proposed Sable Gas Pipeline Project from the perspective of Environmentally Induced Illness/Chemical Sensitivity, Asthma and allergy, February, 2007. On-line at www.geocities.com/RainForest/6847/report1.html.

Combustion Gases in Your Home — Things You Should Know About Combustion Spillage. Are Combustion

Gases Spilling Into Your Home? Order from the Canada Mortgage and Housing Corporation, Suite 1000, 700 Montreal Rd. Ottawa, ON K1A 0P7. By phone: (800) 668-2642. On-line: http://www.cmhc-schl.gc.ca/en/co/maho/yohoyohe/inaiqu/inaiqu_004.cfm

RESOURCES

Combustible Gas Sniffers
The TIF Model 8800A Combustible Gas Detector is recommended to check for gas leaks. *Professional Equipment.* Phone: (800) 334-9291.
Website: http://www.professionalequipment.com

Power Vents
To add a power vent to an existing gas water heater to prevent back-drafting of combustion gases. Mounts on the outside of the building and pulls the combustion gas from the appliance through the outside wall utilizing negative pressure.
Phone: (252) 523-8255
Web Site: http://www.ddchem.com/swg-vent_kits.htm

Tank-less hot Water Heaters
Most brands of hot water heaters now make a tank-less, electric or power vented gas unit. Bosch is a brand that has been around a long time. To learn more about tank-less water heaters see http://www.bosch.com.mx/content/language2/html/2460.htm and http://www.bosch.com.mx/content/language2/html/2492.htm.

END NOTES

1. Baker-Laporte, Paula, Erica Elliot, M.D., and John Banta. *Prescriptions for a Healthy House.* New Society Publishers, 2001, p. 6.
2. Aerotech Labs. *IAQ Tech Tip on Carbon Monoxide, 2005.* http://www.aerotechpk.com/Resources/TechtipDetails.aspx?i=13&t=Product (cited online February 2007).
3. Canada Mortgage and Housing Corporation. *Clean Guide.* 1993, p. 2.
4. Dadd, Lynn. *Home Safe Home.* Penguin Putnam Inc., New York, 1997.
5. Zamm, Alfred V., M.D. *Why Your House May Endanger Your Health.* Simon and Shuster, New York, 1980, p. 23.

8 - WIRING

WHAT IS IT?

The presence of electrical wiring in homes and offices produce what are called electro-magnetic fields (EMF). When the power is on, the wiring is energized. Anything that is plugged in, even if it is turned off has an electric field close to it. When something is turned on, current flows and a magnetic field is created also.

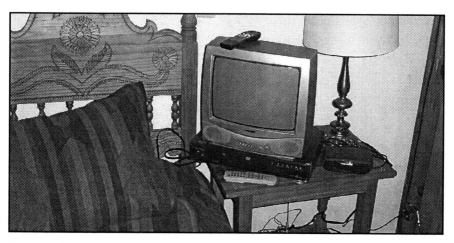

The most significant thing affecting you sleep may be the electric and magnetic fields emitted by the clock radio or other electronic gadgets close to the bed.

WHAT CAN IT DO TO ME?

A voltage is induced on the body from house wiring similar to a battery. You can measure the voltage induced on your body from household wiring using a multi-meter available at any hardware store.

The biological effects have largely been ignored in the press, possibly because all the media focus has been on power lines causing cancer. Stress, difficulty concentrating, and sleeping problems are associated with EMF. Laboratory studies have found EMFs to cause changes in hormones including melatonin, biorhythms, brain activity, heart rate, and alterations in the immune system.[1]

Linked to electromagnetic field exposure are:

- Insomnia and sleep disorders

- Fatigue

- Headaches

- Muscle cramps and menstruation disorders

- Nerve problems, irritability

- Attention Deficit Disorder (ADD)

- Allergy aggravation.

Studies suggest that electromagnetic fields may promote the development of existing cancers even if they don't initiate cancer.[2]

WHERE IS IT?

Electromagnetic fields are present near wiring, electrical outlets, extension cords, lights, appliances, and anything that is plugged in to an electrical outlet. The closer one is to wiring the more they are potentially effected.

Electric fields come from the wiring inside walls. Most walls have wiring in them that coincidentally happens to be at the height of your head when you are lying in bed.

Electricians commonly make wiring errors that can cause a higher exposure indoors than from standing under power lines. Results of a recent study at K-12 schools indicate that wiring errors may be a more important source of exposure than power lines.[3] The most common wiring errors are tying the white, "neutral" wires from different circuits together, and using the wrong type of wiring for 3-way switches.

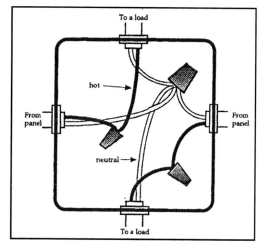

The most common type of wiring error — neutrals (white wires) from different circuits tied together. Reproduced from: *Tracing EMF's in Building Wiring and Grounding.* Courtesy, Karl Riley.

GET RID OF IT!!!

Most scientists agree that electromagnetic fields affect us biologically and that prudent avoidance is in our best interest. You don't have to go back to living in a cave. It is very easy to minimize exposure in rooms where a lot of time is spent including the bedroom.

Use a battery-operated alarm clock. Many sleeping disorders have been solved by replacing electric-powered alarm clocks with battery powered ones.

Avoid placing the head of the bed against a wall on the other side of which is an appliance, fuse box, TV, or computer.

Remove as many electrical cords and devices from around the bed as possible. It is reported that many troubling conditions—such as children wetting the bed, babies who wake frequently, and adults who are insomniacs—are relieved of symptoms when this is done.[4]

Do not use an electric blanket or put it on a timer to go off after you fall asleep.

Keep your distance. Exposure decreases with distance. An electric space heater for example, will produce a large field close by. Three feet away is good; six feet is ideal.

The ultimate way to reduce EMF exposure and possibly get a good night sleep may be to shut off the power to the bedroom at night. This may seem radical but it's the quickest way to tell how EMFs may be affecting your sleep. It is also worth the trouble to just move the location of the bed for a few weeks and see if a difference is noted.

If you want to check for wiring errors caused by an electrician you will need a gauss meter. Turn on all the lights. While standing in the center of the room, have someone else go around and turn on and off each light switch. Any change in the reading on the meter indicates a wiring error. When solving problems, it helps to speak to electricians in a language they can understand. Tell them there is "net current" from a wiring error. Net current is prohibited by the National Electric Code.[5]

Lesson Learned

Eight years ago, a family remodeled a beautiful and spacious house in an expensive neighborhood near the California coast. This family has a very healthy diet, and the mother is extremely heath conscious, but one of her two sons has diabetes. There are no factors, including family history, that explain his illness.

Wondering if there could be any environmental factors responsible for her son's disease, she ordered a comprehensive environmental assessment of the house. The investigation turned up none of the usual culprits associated with an unhealthy home. The house was dry and free of mold and furnished with non-toxic materials.

What the investigation did find were high levels of magnetic fields throughout the house. The level in the boys' bedrooms was 7mG (cancer and biological effects have been associated with levels greater than 2mg). These were found to be from wiring errors made by the electrician during the remodel eight years ago.

After this discovery, an electrician spent four days locating and correcting all the problems. This included making corrections in many places where three-way switches were installed. Three-way switches allow us to turn on and off lights using switches from different sides of the room.

In addition to fixing the wiring problems, the son's bed was moved (it had been near the fuse box) and the family turned off the Wi-Fi at night. Within two weeks the mother reported her son with diabetes was improving. This supported studies that show diabetes might be caused by high electromagnetic fields, especially when there are no other factors to account for the disease.

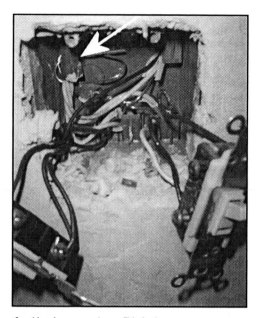

One big wire nut syndrome. This is the most common type of wiring error that may result in high levels of magnetic fields, sometimes as large as those found under power lines outdoors. The neutrals (white wires) from different circuits have been tied together.

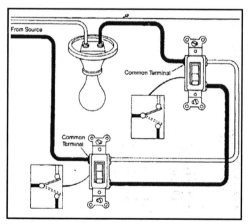

Bad advice — this drawing found in a how-to-do book on electrical wiring incorrectly shows how to wire three-way switches. The black wire by itself on the left side of the picture will cause an elevated magnetic field. It should be paired with a white wire everywhere it goes. Wiring like this drawing is against code.

Electromagnetic fields show up where we least expect them. When I first became trained to test for magnetic fields, I noticed power lines close to my house and was surprised to find that my house was not affected by the power lines. The fields emitted dropped off quickly with distance.

I then went to a friend's house where the power lines are buried under ground. The level was low outside, but inside the meter jumped when we turned on a ceiling fan. When the house was built, the electrician didn't use the right type of wiring for the three-way switches. Short of ripping the wiring out of the walls, the only way to fix the problem was to have only one switch for the fan.

When you are remodeling or having a new home built, it is important to talk to the electrician and make it clear that he follow the National Electric Code and avoid these problems.

SUGGESTED READING

For a detailed synopsis of the major studies done regarding the potential heath effects of electromagnetic fields, read *Warning: the electricity around you may be hazardous to your health*, by Sugarman, Ellen, 2nd Edition, Simon & Shuster, 1992, Appendix A.

For detailed explanation of wiring errors made by electricians and how to resolve them, read *Tracing EMFs in Building Wiring and Grounding* by Karl Riley. The book or DVD can be ordered through Magnetic Sciences at (800) 749-9873.

Another good text for electricians and homeowners is *Silencing the Fields; A Practical Guide to Reducing AC Magnetic Fields* by Ed Leeper. Can be ordered online at http://www.silencingthefields.com or by phone (303) 442-3773.

RESOURCES

A gauss meter is needed to measure magnetic fields from power lines and wiring errors. *Dr. Gauss* is an affordable unit. For those who want something more accurate and less susceptible to interference, the *F.W. Bell Model 4080* Tri axial. Less EMF also rents this meter.

Less EMF
Phone: (888) 537-7363
Web site: www.lessemf.com

Professional Equipment
Phone: (800) 334-9291
Web site: www.professionalequipment.com

To find a professional trained in testing and consulting, call the **International Institute for Baubiologie & Ecology (IBE)**. The institute also offers an online training course and seminars. Phone: (727) 461-4371.
Web site: www.bau-biologieusa.com

Mike Holt
Mike Holt is nationally recognized as one of America's most knowledgeable electrical trainers. He has expert knowledge of the National Electrical Code and helping electricians understand it. Phone: (888) NEC-Code, (888) 632-2633
Web site: www.mikeholt.com

END NOTES

1. National Institute of Environmental Health Services and U.S. Department of Energy. *Questions and Answers About EMF, Electric and Magnetic Fields Associated with the Use of Electric Power*. U.S. Government Printing Office, Washington, D.C., January 1995, p.23.
2. Ibid.
3. Adams, Jack, Samuel Bitler, and Karl Riley. "Importance of Addressing National Electric Code Violations That Result in Unusual Exposure to 60 HZ Magnetic Fields." *Bioelectromagnetics*, 25:102-106 (2004).

See also: Janie Magruder. "School loses magnetic hot spot." *The Mesa Tribune*, January, 1991.
4. Thompson, Athena. *Homes that Heal and those that don't, How your home may be harming your family's health*. New Society Publishers, 2004, p. 112.
5. *The National Electric Code 2002*, Article 300.3 and Article 310-4, "Conductors of the Same Circuits."

9 - MYSTERY TOXINS

WHAT IS IT?

Mystery toxins are things that are affecting your health but you cannot identify exactly what they are or where they are coming from. Some people are bothered by quantities that don't seem significant.

Mystery toxins can be associated with mold or water damage. Mold spores may have dried up and fragmented into small pieces that are undetectable by scientific testing. The particles nonetheless are still present, allergenic, and affect heath.

Mystery toxins can be insulation, rodent droppings and other kinds of allergens, dust particles, odors, and chemicals.

WHAT CAN IT DO TO ME?

Mystery toxins can cause a variety of health symptoms similar to mold exposure or the other hazards on the Top Ten list. When people complain about heath problems caused by their home or office, and investigators can't figure out why they call it a *sick building*. Common symptoms of living in a sick building include headache, fatigue, and eyes, nose, and throat irritation.

WHERE IS IT?

The sources of mystery toxins are usually not out in the open and clearly visible. They penetrate the living space from inside wall-cavities, below the flooring, and above the ceiling. Often they are brought in from the air-conditioning and heating system.

It is common practice to use wall and ceiling cavities as the return air ducts. The furnace and air conditioning pull air from these walls or ceiling into the air you are breathing. Building cavities should never be used as return ducts.

Sometimes wall cavities being used as air ducts have fiberglass insulation in them. This is done to minimize noise created by air movement through them. It is not necessary if ducts are designed properly.

Typically, ducts leak between 10-15%, and 25-30% leakage is not uncommon.[1] This means that if the ducts are in the ceiling or crawlspace, some of the air you breathe will contain air from the ceiling or crawlspace.

Many problems are caused by basements and crawlspaces. Warm air rises like hot air in a chimney. Air from the crawlspace or basement is sucked through cracks in the floor and up into the living space.

The grill covering the opening under the furnace has been removed to take this picture. Air is supposed to be sucked from the hallway into the furnace. It will also be sucked from inside the wall cavity under the furnace. This may not sound too bad until you look inside. Rodent droppings and urine and concrete and saw dust are common.

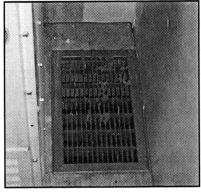

Sometimes with gas heaters there is a vent on the floor in the closet that is open directly to the crawlspace or basement. This is a bad idea. It is done to provide air for the gas to burn. It also allows unhealthy air to get upstairs and into the duct work. This can be covered up if a hole is cut in the door and the vent put there or a duct for venting is run up from the closet through the roof. Check local building code.

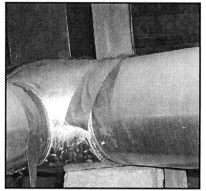

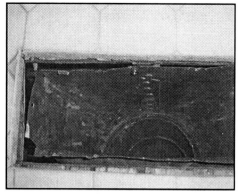

A study found 200 good uses for duct tape and only one bad one — sealing ducts. Most furnace ducts leak, potentially pulling in air from crawlspaces, attics and where ever else the ducts go. Use mastic instead.

Air gaps around a heating duct in the floor. The gaps allow for air from the crawlspace or basement to get into the air upstairs.

GET RID OF IT!!!

Investigate and Clean the Air-conditioning System

Studies have shown that investigating the heating and air-conditions systems is capable of resolving 80% of complaints related to the indoor environment. [2] If you have a forced-air heating or air-conditioning system, pull the access panels off and look inside. Change the filter. Clean the air-conditioning drain pan. If there is fibrous insulation inside it replace it or seal it with aluminum foil and metal tape.

Air-conditioners are huge de-humidifiers. Water condenses inside them. Slime mold and bacteria can grow if the pan is not draining properly. Inspect the system in the summer when it's running and make sure it's draining properly.

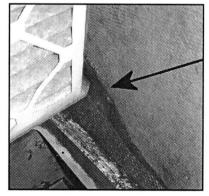

Mold growing on the inside lining of an air conditioner in a public building. The drain pain was overflowing allowing water to lap onto the filter.

Increase Ventilation

One study found that 70% of sick buildings simply have inadequate flows of fresh outside air.[3] By simply increasing the amount of fresh air, people felt well and complaints were solved. Ventilation can be as simple as opening windows. If you can't open a window because you have pollen allergies, install a HEPA filter on the heating and cooling system that brings in outdoor air and filters it.

Commercial buildings have outdoor, fresh-air intakes attached to the heating and cooling system. Sadly, they are often closed to save on utility bills. The number one reason for complaints in office buildings and schools is that the outdoor air-intake has been completely closed off.[4]

Ask maintenance to locate the fresh air-intake and open it. It is often on the roof, covered with a screen to keep birds out. You cannot have too much fresh air.

Avoid using wall and ceiling cavities as ductwork

At home, take the grill that covers the furnace return vent off and look inside. You may find yourself looking into a wall or ceiling cavity with lots of dust and debris left over from construction, rodent droppings, and fiberglass insulation.

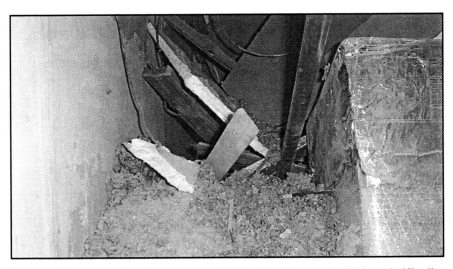

Dust and debris above the ceiling tiles in a commercial building. The foil box on the right is an air-chiller. Air is pulled from the ceiling cavity into the chiller and blown into the office space below.

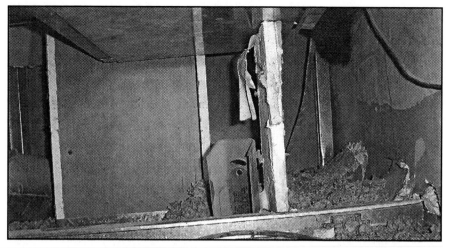

Dust and debris above the suspended ceiling tiles in a commercial building. The insulation is rock wool, a possible carcinogen. What is it doing here?

In your office, pop one of the ceiling tiles. You will be looking at the vast empty space and dust above the suspended ceiling. It's difficult to clean all the dust that accumulates on top of these tiles. They should all be taken down and cleaned. Older tiles may contain asbestos. Caution is required.

The ultimate, healthy alternative in both home and office is to run ductwork directly to the heating or cooling system instead of using the ceiling or wall cavities as ductwork.

Seal Ductwork

If ductwork is in the attic, above the ceiling, in the crawlspace or basement, seal the seams and joints with mastic. Apply it with a paintbrush. Duct tape should not be used to seal ducts. Duct tape dries up, falls off, and rots within a few years.

Keep it in the crawlspace or basement

The ultimate way to keep odors and nasties out of the living space from the crawlspace is to treat crawl spaces as mini-basements. This means pouring a concrete slab and heating the crawlspace or basement to 65 degrees in the winter.

The next best thing to do is to create a vacuum in the crawlspace. Install fans in a few of the existing vents that are used to ventilate the crawlspace to the outside. Seal up the remaining vents so that a vacuum is created when the fans are running. If the air pressure in the crawlspace is maintained lower than upstairs, air will not flow from the crawlspace to the upstairs through cracks in the floor.

Install a plastic vapor barrier on top of the soil in the crawlspace. The completed project would look like a giant swimming pool liner that includes the ground and the foundation walls. This is more effective if gravel, perforated pipes, and a fan are used to suck air out from underneath the vapor barrier, similar to what is used for radon mitigation.

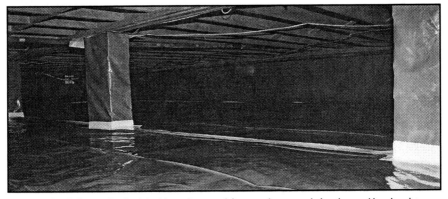

A properly installed vapor barrier (plastic) on the ground in a crawl space seals in odors, mold and moisture.
Photo Courtesy: Vapor Free, Inc.

Get some expanding foam in an aerosol can. Go into the crawlspace and seal around any gaps in the flooring around pipes, wiring and other things penetrating the floor. Pay particular attention to sealing around the holes cut out for ductwork vents and around plumbing under kitchen and bathroom sinks.

Preaching to the Choir

Another perfectly clean house. Hours spent investigating for clues. What was my client allergic to? She had spent a small fortune furnishing the home with healthy furniture and carpet. She used non-fragrant laundry soap and cleaning supplies. I felt like I was preaching to the choir.

The only thing I could suspect was the attached garage on the bottom floor, under the living room. There were cans of gas stored in the garage. There were stairs that led from the living room to the garage. It was probable that gas fumes were leaking upstairs.

A combustible gas meter is used to check for gas. It's a relative sensor. You turn it on outside then go inside and it will start beeping if it detects gas.

Sure enough, indoors it beeped. But in the garage there was less beeping. The sensor is also sensitive to humidity. In Florida they would say I was crazy. But in the southwest, the humidity can be less than 6%, and the instrument was responding to a change in humidity. It meant the house was too tightly sealed.

Because the client was allergic to juniper pollen, she kept the windows closed year-round. The house was air tight with no ventilation. She really needed some fresh air. In her efforts to create a healthy home and eliminate pollen, she had sealed herself into an environment that wouldn't let any other toxins out. Remember the rain barrel effect? The solution was simple: install an outdoor air intake on the roof next to the air-conditioning with a HEPA filter to filter the pollen out but let the fresh air in.

SUGGESTED READING

Lstiburek, Joseph P., Eng., *Builder's Guide*, Energy Efficient Building Association.
Phone: (952) 881-3048
Web site: www.buildingscience.com

May, Jeffrey C., *My House is Killing Me!* John Hopkins University Press, Baltimore, Maryland, 2001.

Thompson, Athena, *Homes that Heal (and those that don't): How your home may be harming your family's health*, New Society Publishers, 2004.

RESOURCES

Power Vents for Crawlspace Ventilation
Eliminator® Foundation Vent Fan
Phone: (252) 523-8255
http://www.ddchem.com/Crawlspace-fan.htm

Crawl Space Ventilator 110 CFM
R.E. Williams
Phone: (661)775-5979
Web Site: www.rewci.com/crspve110cfm.html

Vapor Barriers for Crawlspaces
Vapor Free, Inc.
Phone: (615) 867-0422
Web Site: www.vaporfree.com

END NOTES

1. Lstiburek, Joseph. "Heating, Ventilating, Air Conditioning, and Air Quality Problems." *The Healthy School Handbook*. National Education Association Professional Library publication, Washington, D.C., 1995, p. 93.
2. Hansen, Shirley J., Ph.D. *Managing Indoor Air Quality*. The Fairmont Press, Lilburn, GA, 1991, p. 181, 207.
3. Kail, Konrad, M.D. Allergy Free, An Alternative Medicine Definitive Guide. Alternative Medicine.com, Tiburon, California, 2000, pg. 142.
4. *The Healthy School Handbook*, p. 65.
5. Ibid., p. 65.
6. Lstiburek, Joseph, P.Eng. *Builder's Guide, Hot-Dry and Mixed-Dry Climates*. Energy Efficient Building Association, Minneapolis, MN, 1998, p. 258. See Chapter 9. It covers air handlers and duct work with good illustrations on how to seal duct work and install heating and air-conditioning systems for good indoor air quality and energy efficiency.
7. *The Healthy School Handbook*, p. 93.

10 - STRESS

Have you ever been stressed out at work and gotten a pimple? Moved to a big city and suddenly became allergic to something that never bothered you before?

Stress affects the body in very real, physical ways including the immune and hormonal systems. Stress can lower one's threshold to allergens and mystery toxins.

One study surveyed 2,160 employees in 67 office buildings with no recognized environmental problems. The researches found a relationship between office workers who reported that the building was *sick* and those who reported having high levels of stress.[1] Job category and job satisfaction, poor management, and boring work influence and lower people's complaint thresholds. [2]

Of another study the author reports, *"Sick building* syndrome may be wrongly named—symptoms appear to be due less to physical conditions than to working environments characterized by poor psychosocial conditions. We are not making claims that buildings don't matter. There certainly could be buildings which do have physical properties that are very bad, but for the general workforce, job stress, and job demands seem to have a bigger impact."[3]

GET RID OF IT

You may not be able to change what's going on around you but you can choose how you react. Don't worry about things you can't control. Don't sweat the small stuff.

Language is the most important factor.[4] Listen to what you are saying to yourself. Your subconscious is powerful. Whatever you tell yourself you are programming yourself into believing. What if you are wrong?

When you catch yourself thinking about something that doesn't feel good, stop. Say, "Cancel, clear, delete," and choose a new thought. No matter what is going on around you, you always have the power to choose your own thoughts.

OLD THOUGHT	NEW THOUGHT
I can't.	I could. I choose not to.
	No thank you.
	I am...(state what you are doing or can do)
I have to.	I have a choice.
	I choose to...
	I am...instead
I don't know.	I don't have enough information.
	I am seeking clarity on that.
	I'd love to know the answer - I'll find out.

Suggestions for up-grading your language to program your mind for success. Excepts from the book: NLP: Transforming Your Life Through Language by Gary De Rodriguez, Life Design International.

Imagine how someone you look up to, perhaps a favorite movie star, would handle him or herself in the same situation. How would they talk? How would they act? Imagine yourself with these qualities.

Visualize a color that will transform the current situation into what you desire. Feel the color penetrating every cell in your body.

When you are feeling stressed take a break and go for a walk. A short morning walk before the office helps put the mind and body at ease.

You can boost your immune system and level of tolerance to stress by taking care of yourself, eating right, resting, and getting some exercise.

Avoid socializing with people who talk negatively. You get more of what ever you focus your attention on. Stop thinking about what you don't want. Think about what you do want.

Most people, if you ask them, cannot tell you what it is they do want. What is it that you want? Consider what the world will look like and how it will feel when you have it. What will be different? What will be the same? What is stopping you from having what you want? Don't answer this question until you have fully considered it.

Now, how do you know?

TOXIC STRESS

Between my careers as an engineer and an indoor environmental consultant, I was a handyman. I would do just about any type of work, not realizing the potential harm I was doing to myself.

One time I found myself very fatigued. That by itself was not unexpected. I had been working a lot of hours, from early morning until late at night. But I had blood in my stool and was so tired I just wanted to lie on the couch all day.

During the previous days I had been cutting railroad ties with a gas-powered chain saw to build a retaining wall. Railroad ties contain creosote, a toxic wood preservative known as coal tar. It's these chemicals that make railroad ties last forever and not grow mold. God knows what I was breathing in the big cloud of smoke that surrounded me as the chain saw struggled to cut through the wood, burning it.

My doctor took blood tests and diagnosed me with anemia, one of the main symptoms of creosote poisoning. Even then, I suspected that there is an emotional aspect to every disease. I could just feel it. My doctor told me I had low blood counts and needed iron shots. My gut told me it was emotional. Were it not for what was going on in my heart and in my head at the time, I know I could have sustained the abuse I was giving my body with the creosote.

I took the iron shots. I ate a diet rich in foods high in vitamin B and iron and took supplements to help my body grow more blood cells. But I knew that until I addressed the emotional aspect of the illness I might not get better, or at least not be fully back to the strength and stamina I had before.

Louise Hay, a well-know author of self-help books, has a list of physical aliments and what she believes are the emotional issues associated with them. Reading the list can be kind of like a horoscope: for any given ailment, what you read seems to apply to your life in some way. Of anemia, it states. "A yes-but attitude, fear of life, and not feeing good enough." Of fatigue it says, "Resistance, boredom, lack of love for what one does."

To me this seemed true. I was unfulfilled working as a handyman. It was not my bliss and I was wondering what to do next. I was also in an unhappy relationship. When I addressed these issues I got better, my anemia went away, and I was able to go hiking again without feeling fatigued. It was the combination of removing myself from further exposure to toxins, taking the stuff my doctor gave me to boost my immune system, and embracing the new that healed me.

SUGGESTED READING

Hay, Louise L. You Can Heal Your Life, Hay House, Carlsbad, CA, 1984.

Dwoskin, Hale. The Sedona Method, Your Keys to Lasting Happiness, Success, Peace and Emotional Well-being, 2003.

RESOURCES

The Sedona Method
While in Sedona, Arizona, I met a rock star who was attending one the Sedona Method's two day seminars. He said, "You know Dan, there's a lot of New Age sh*t in this town. But this [Sedona Method] really gets to the bottom of things." During the workshop he was so inspired he finished writing a song. He played it to the group during the seminar. It brought tears to their eyes. I don't think it was the kind of song typical of his rock band. Jack Canfield, co-author of the Chicken Soup for the Soul, also recommends the Sedona Method.
Sedona Training Associates
Phone: (928) 282-3522
Web site: www.sedona.com

Naka-Ima
Workshops with techniques similar to the Sedona Method. Based on the principle that being honest is the surest path to joy, success, and well-being.
Portland, Oregon. Phone: (503) 804-6086
Web site: www.nakaima.org

Life Design International
Customized corporate training programs; Individual coaching sessions
Gary de Rodriguez, Founder
Phone: (505) 982-1980
Web site: lifedesignInternational.com

END NOTES

1. Ooi, P.L. "Sick Building Syndrome: An emerging Stress-Related Disorder?" International Journal of Epidemiology, Volume 26, No. 6, pp. 1243-1249.
2. Macher, Janet, Ed. Bioaerosols: Assessment and Control. American Conference of Governmental Industrial Hygienists, Cincinnati, Ohio, 1999, p. 3-9.
3. Green Building Press, Is Stress A Factor In 'Sick Building Syndrome? http://www.newbuilder.co.uk/news/NewsFullStory.asp?ID=1283 (cited online April 2006).
4. In conversation with Gary Rodriguez, President of Life Design International, at a Nero-Linguistic Programming Practitioner training seminar in 2005, Rodriguez stated that language is the most important factor in determining if people regress to previous states of mind after having made changes in their beliefs. Jack Canfield, co-author of the Chicken Soup for the Soul series recommends Neuro-linguistic Programming (The Success Principles. Harper Collins, 2005, pg 262).

RECOMMENDATIONS

Vacuum Cleaners

A HEPA type vacuum cleaner is recommended. HEPA means High Efficiency Particle Aresstance. HEPA products remove 99.97% of particles greater 0.3 microns in size. If you don't have a good HEPA vacuum, the small, unseen particles are blown back out of the bag into the air. Sometimes you can smell them.

Nowadays, you can find HEPA vacuums at just about every department store. Most of these are not HEPA. Many are junk. Manufactures are not required by law to test their products and there are no consumer protection laws regarding what can be labeled a HEPA vacuum.

How to find a good HEPA Vacuum cleaner

- Look for one with the filter after the motor. The filter should be the last thing that air goes by before exiting the vacuum. If the motor is the last thing, particles from the motor bushings will be emitted into the air.

- Gaskets that prevent air from bypassing the filter.

- Ask. Ask the store clerk for a demonstration with a laser particle counter. Hold the particle counter up to the exhaust of the vacuum while it is running. It should read nearly zero. This is the only way to be certain a vacuum cleaner is HEPA.

Our testing with a laser particle counter has found a few brands that are truly HEPA: Nilfisk, Miele and Sebo (model with the HEPA type "S-Class" filtration micro filter). Miele also sells a non-HEPA vacuum, which performs better than most other brands claiming to be HEPA. This is probably due to the gasket design that prevents air from going around the filter. Water and bag-less filters often do not test HEPA.

To locate a dealer near you:
Miele (800) 843-7231. On the web at www.miele.com
Nilfisk (610) 647 6420. On the web at http://nilfisk.com

If your vacuum cleaner dealer does not have a particle counter suggest they get one:
The Particle Scan Pro by IQAir
Web site: http://www.iqair.us
Phone: (877) 715-4247

If you don't have a good vacuum cleaner there are some things you can do to protect your health and those around you when vacuuming:

- Schedule cleaning when no one is around and when you can leave immediately after vacuuming

- Open the windows

- Turn on an air purifier.

Never allow hired help to use their vacuum cleaner. You don't know where it's been.

Furnace Filters - What's Not Recommended

Washable filters
Washable filters are either electronic or use static electricity. Many new homes have electronic air cleaners. Builders install them because they are cheap and

it makes it seem like a healthy home.

If you have an electronic air cleaner you may think you're lucky because you don't need to replace filters. You simply wash them. When these filters are tested using a laser particle counter they are very poor at removing small dust particles. Dust may collect on these filters, but only the big stuff.

The washable polyester and polypropylene filters test so poorly that the manufacturers rate them using an arrestance scale rather than a MERV scale. This sounds like a reasonable test except for the fact that about 5% of all dust particles are big, heavy, and responsible for about 95% of the total weight of the dust. The other 95% of particles are small and weigh nearly nothing but have the most potential to affect your health and pass right through these filters.

Stock filters

The typical throwaway filter that came with your furnace is not intended to clean the air. It is designed to protect the moving parts in the furnace. As a rule of thumb, if you hold the filter up to the light and can see though it, dust will pass through it.

Ultra-Violet Light (UV)

Some companies sell ultra-violet lights to put in your furnace to prevent mold and bacteria. This is a waste of money. Mold spores are relatively unaffected by ultraviolet light.[1] Mold has a tough shell to protect it against sunlight. Even if mold could be killed, ultra-violet light does nothing to neutralize allergens and toxins on the cell walls of mold spores.

UV light is effective in killing bacteria and viruses. There is, however, no evidence that indoor exposure to most human-shed bacteria results in specific health complaints or allergies.[2] Bacteria are present everywhere. They are part of the body's natural micoflora. Pathogenic bacteria are not normally present in residential living spaces.

If harmful bacteria are present, UV-light is not the answer. It's not enough to just kill bacteria. You must find and correct the source otherwise you will continue be exposed to toxins from bacteria called endotoxins. When the cell walls of dead bacteria desiccate, fragments containing toxins become air-borne.

The only practical application of UV-light may be in air-conditioning when it shines directly on the cooling coils. This should not be necessary if the air-conditioning drain pan is draining properly.

Antimicrobial Coatings

This is unnecessary and ineffective. Most antimicrobial coatings are referred to as "bound" because the chemicals in them bind to the surface of the filter. As the filter becomes dirty, dirt acts as a barrier between the treated filter and potentially harmful organisms. This eliminates the anti-microbial effectiveness.[3] Mold cannot grow without moisture. If a filter is getting wet something is seriously wrong that requires immediate attention. Mold will grow on the dust.

Air Filter Guide[4]

| | | PARTICLE SIZE | | |
	Less than 0.3 microns (μ)	0.3 to 1 microns	1 to 3 microns	3 to 10 microns
	Smoke	Cat allergens	Aspergillus mold (3.5 μ)	Skin flakes
	Smog	Dog allergens		Most molds
	Atmospheric Dust	Dust mites	Penicillium mold (3.3 μ)	Stachybotrys "black mold" (5.7 μ)
	Asbestos	Bacteria	Bacteria	
	Viruses		Lead dust	Pollen
TYPE OF AIR FILTER	**MERV Rating**	**Efficiency**	**Efficiency**	**Efficiency**	**Efficiency**
Ozone Ionizers UV light Stock paper filters	1	0	0	0	<20%
Electrostatic filters	4	0	0	0	<20%
Electronic filters	8	0	0	0	20 – 80%
Allergy reduction paper pleated filters	11	0	0	065-80 % Before installing	085 % Before installing
HEPA	17		99.97% Theoretical Most models 80% to 90 % actual at best.		

 Your body has difficulty removing particles less than 0.5 microns in size. 90% of all particles are less than 0.3 microns.

 Your body's natural defense mechanisms can easily remove particles greater than 3 microns in size.

Furnace Filters - What is Recommended

Disposable Filters

For furnace filters buy a MERV 11 rated filter. The 3M Corporation makes a MERV 11 filter called Filtrete available at most hardware and department stores.

Whole-house Filters

If you want to do better than a MERV 11 then you will have to install a whole-house filter system. A whole-house filter attaches either directly to the furnace or the ductwork.

A HEPA filter will provide the best filtration. Particles that HEPA filters remove better than other filter types include allergens, smoke, pet dander, dust mite allergens, and fine atmospheric dust.

IQAir makes a MERV 16 rated whole-house filter that, although not technically a HEPA filter, removes 95% of particles 0.3 microns in size and is more economical than their whole-house HEPA units.

Whole-House HEPA Filtration Systems

Contact your local heating and cooling contractor for more information.

Product	Manufacturer	Pros	Cons
Guardian Plus (U.S.) HEPA 3000/4000 (Canada)	Broan-NuTone, LLC (Venmar in Canada) P.O. Box 140 Hartford, WI 53027 In U.S.A. call: (800) 558-1711 In Canada call: (877) 896-1119	Good for outdoor air exchange. Has a built in fresh air exchanger that brings air in to the filter while simultaneously exhausting stale air outdoors. Available with heat or energy recovery option.	No carbon filter. HEPA filter appears to be thinner than other brands. Reported to not filter as effective as 99.97% at 0.3 microns[9]. Made of plastic.
HEPA Shield 600HS Larger models available for commercial buildings	Pure Air Systems, Inc. 1325 Church Street Clayton, IN 46118 Phone: (317) 291-4341 (800) 869-8025 pureairsystems.com	A thick HEPA filter. Bigger is better? 5 lb carbon filter. Optional carbon/ alumina /zeolite blend for removing formaldehyde in new homes.	Does not come with a fresh air exchanger. A fresh air intake duct can be added.

Contact your local heating and cooling contractor for more information.

Product	Manufacturer	Pros	Cons
Perfect 16	IQAir http://www.iqair.us 1-877-715-4 AIR (247)	Designed so that there is minimal air resistance and no fan or motor needed. Optional carbon filter. Probably the highest filtration efficiency possible with out going to a HEPA filter. Cost less than the IQAir Clean Zone	No fresh air exchange. Not technically a HEPA filter, a MERV 16 rated filter. Removes 95% of particles 0.3 microns and larger.
IQAir Clean Zone	IQAir http://www.iqair.us 1-877-715-4 AIR (247)	Filters down to .003 micron (virus) size particles. Possibly the best air purification system in the world.	No carbon filter. Expensive.

Whichever brand you get, install and connect an outdoor-air-intake to it. The duct to bring in outdoor air is similar to a dryer duct. It should connect from the outside to the intake of the filter so that the outdoor air is filtered before being distributed in your home or office.

The most common outdoor allergen is pollen.[5] For those allergic to pollen, installing a whole-house HEPA filter with an outdoor air intake essentially replicates being able to open the windows for fresh air without getting any pollen inside.

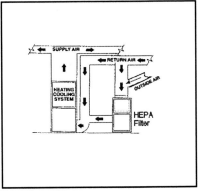

An outdoor air intake attached to a HEPA filter on the furnace. This filters out pollen and other air pollution before supplying fresh air indoors. Courtesy: Pure Air Systems, Inc.

Room Air Purifiers

Even if you think you don't need a room air purifier it can be beneficial to have one around. What do you do if there is a bad air quality day, perhaps a forest fire that has blown smoke your way?

There are two primary considerations in finding a good air purifier. First, it should not introduce anything new into the air. Second, it should clean the air.

What's Not Recommended

Ozone and ion generators

These introduce something new into the air. Ozone is a respiratory irritant. Repeated exposure may permanently scar lung tissue, worsen bronchitis, emphysema, and asthma.[6] Exposure to ozone may make one as much as three times more susceptible to other allergens.[7] There are class action lawsuits against the manufactures of ozone generating devices including Sharper Image and Alpine/EcoQuest.

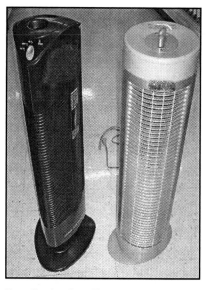

Some people swear they feel better with an ozone air purifier running in their home. As these machines do virtually nothing to remove small particles such as molds and pollen from the air, it is likely that the ozone is reacting with their body. Perhaps their reaction is due to the fact that ozone diminishes the sense of smell.

Many *filter-less* air purifiers generate ozone. Some make it on purpose; others produce it unintentionally. Instead of paper filters, these have metal plates that are supposed to be cleaned periodically. When electricity used to charge the metal plates reacts with oxygen, ozone is produced.

There are applications where ozone is effective. Ozone has been shown to be effective in smoke damage to alleviate odors. The amount of ozone required is hazardous and the building must be vacated while the ozone machines are running. It is not completely effective. Ozone only reacts with what is at the surface and odors often migrate to the surface later causing the smoke odors to come back. Ozone may damage contents in a home including rubber and synthetic furniture.[8]

Room Air Purifiers - What is Recommended

HEPA Filters

Buy an air purifier with a HEPA filter. Some complain about the time and expense of changing filters. If there were an easier way, the government, hospitals, and computer chip manufactures would not be spending money on HEPA filters.

Some people don't like the noise that the fan in a HEPA air purifier makes. You don't need it all of the time, just when you notice poor air quality or that you're waking up in the morning congested. A compromise that seems to work for a lot of people is to turn the air purifier on high speed when you first get home then turn it down later. If the air purifier is in the bedroom, turn it on high about one hour before you go into the bedroom. It may be possible to turn it off at night.

It can be overwhelming trying to choose from all the makes and models of HEPA filter air purifiers on the market. Manufactures compete with each other, make claims, and cite specifications of being better in various ways. Most of these are not supported by accurate testing methods. Consumer review publications are not the best way to get un-biased information.

The only sure way to assess the effectiveness of an air cleaner is know that it has been tested using a laser particle counter. There should be nearly zero particles coming out of the unit when it is running. The only company that tests every unit that it sells using a laser particle counter is the Swiss IQAir. Every IQAir air purifier sold is tested. Each unit comes with a certificate with the actual test results.

Air purifiers should also have something to remove chemicals and odors. HEPA filters only removes dust particles. Most brands have a filter to absorb odors and chemicals in addition to a HEPA filter. Many have a pre-filter made out of a thin, black, polyester lining that contains carbon. This is not sufficient. There should be a granulated mixture that includes a binder such as activated alumina impregnated with potassium permanganate. Potassium permanganate is a dark purple substance that is a powerful oxidizing agent for gas and odor control. We have found that clients, even those who didn't think they needed chemical and odor removal, felt better if they had it. The IQAir *Health Pro Plus* has both HEPA and odor removal filters.

A Fine White Dust

Everything in the bedroom was covered with a very fine layer of white dust. If you took your finger and ran it across the top of the book case shelf, TV, or bedpost, you would find it everywhere in the bedroom.

As usual, the client was worried it might be mold. So we tested for mold. I inspected the crawlspace below the bedroom and walked the roof looking for problems. Nothing. And the rest of the house was quite clean, with no signs of this white powder. I inspected the indoors high and low for sources of the white dust.

In the Mike's bedroom there was one of those air purifiers with metal plates that you are supposed to clean. Air purifiers that don't have filters normally don't do much to reduce the level of dust indoors. But in this case there seemed to be a lot of the white powder collecting on the metal plates of this poplar brand of machine. So it seemed it might have been helping.

The stuff almost seemed like baby or talcum powder, so I nervously went through Mike's personal hygiene habits and inspected the bathroom adjoining the bedroom for sources of white stuff.

At our wit's end to find a source, I sent a sample to a forensic lab. They used an electron microscope and a long list of other specialized equipment to identify exactly what the white stuff was. It turned out to be a ceramic. And the only source of ceramics turned out to be parts inside the air purifier. The company that manufactures it said the white stuff was from the residue of the humidifier in the bedroom. But a sample of the residue from it was completely different.

The company asked what we wanted. My client, sick in bed from other health problems and not having the energy to pursue the matter any further, only wanted the dust to go away. He didn't care about anything else. We sent the machine back for a refund. I asked the company to replace the carpet in his bedroom since I didn't think it could be cleaned, but we never heard back.

RESOURCES

Healthy Living Spaces
Visit the website: HealthyLivingSpaces.com
Call: toll-free (877) 992-9904
HEPA room air purifiers, whole-house filters & vacuum cleaners

IQAir
The Health Pro Plus model includes a filter for both particulates and chemicals & odors.
Phone: (800) 500-4247
Web site: www.iqair.us

E.L. Foust Co.
The Foust Series 400 is a line of air purifiers with carbon that satisfies many chemically-sensitive
   people. Foust also makes a portable air purifier for autos, the 160AN.
Phone: (800) 353-6878
Web site: www.foustco.com

END NOTES

1. W.J. Kowalski, PE, "Airborne Respiratory Diseases and Mechanical Systems for Control of
    Microbes" *Heating/Piping/Air-Conditioning,* July 1998, p. 46.
2. American Industrial Hygiene Association. Field Guide for the Determination of Biological Con-
    taminants in Environmental Samples, 1996, p. 40.
3. Janet Macher, ed.*Bioaerosols: Assessment and Control.* American Conference of Governmental
    Industrial Hygienists, Cincinnati, Ohio, 1999, p. 16-7.
4. Some information in the Air Filter Guide is adapted from Comparing Various Filters to MERV
    Ratings, and Indoor Air Quality for the 21st Century, the Definitive Guide on Filtration, Ventila-
    tion and Environmental Control, Pure Air Systems Inc., Clayton, Indiana, August 2002, and from
    Table E-1, Application Guidelines, ANSI/ASHRAE standard 52-2.
5. Notes, CIE training course given by Chelsea Group LLC at Restoration Consultants, Sacra-
    mento, CA, June, 2006.
6. Environmental Protection Agency, *Ozone: Good Up High; Bad Nearby,*
    http://epa.gov/oar/oaqps/gooduphigh/bad.html [cited online February 2007].
7. Field Guide for the Determination of Biological Contaminates in Environmental Samples, Amer-
    ican Industrial Hygiene Association, p. 29.
8. Institute of Inspection, Cleaning and Restoration Certification. IICRC S520 Standard and Refer-
    ence Guide for Professional Mold Remediation, 2003., p. 117.
9. Telephone conversations with IQAir Corporation regarding the IQAir MERV16 and Clean
    Zone HEPA filter systems and comparable data to other brands of whole-house HEPA filters.
    July, 2006.

TIPS FOR BUILDING A HEALTHY HOME

Building a new house presents you with a special opportunity to do things in ways that will support the health of your family for years to follow. The following are the essentials. Detailed specifications are available by contacting the publisher.

If you have the opportunity, consider building a natural home instead of a conventionally built, *stick* house with drywall. Natural homes simply feel better to be in. Spend some time in a natural home so you can experience this for yourself before making a decision.

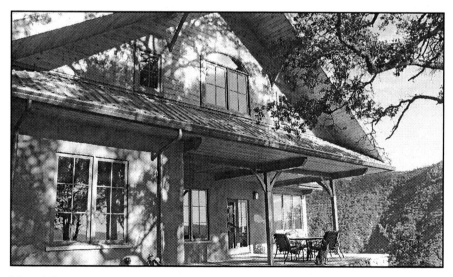

A home built with natural materials. Photo by JT Heater, architect, Nevada City, California.

How much more does it cost to build a natural home? It depends. The cost of a building a natural home may be comparable to building a high-quality, conventional custom home. If you can live with a slightly smaller square footage, money is available to spend on quality materials. An experienced architect and builder may be able to build you a natural home for a price similar to that of a conventional one. Once you live in a natural home you will probably never want to go back to the norm.

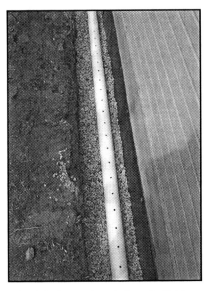

A French Drain: a perforated pipe embedded in gravel, sloped to drain water away from the house.

Big Hat, Big Boots
(Chapter 1: Mold)

No matter what kind of materials you use to build you house, if water penetrates into the interior, mold will grow. There are three design features that help maintain overall low moisture penetration:

- A good roof with an adequate overhang

- A gravel, *French drain* system around the foundation.

- Breathable walls. Water must have a way to get out if it gets in.

Use Dry Wood (Chapter 1: Mold)

Get a moisture meter. Lumber arriving at the job site should be free of mold. The moisture content should be below 10% in most areas. If lumber is damp, don't install it. Send it back.

Drywall (Chapter 1: Mold)

Use DensArmor® Wallboard in bathrooms and kitchens, behind sinks, bathtubs, showers, and dishwashers. It has a fiberglass backing instead of paper. Mold cannot grow on it.

Leave a quarter to half-inch gap above the floor when installing drywall. This prevents water from wicking up the wall and causing mold growth in the event of a flood or plumbing leak. The gap won't be visible after the baseboards are installed.

Termite Control (Chapter 2: Pesticides)

It may be unnecessary to treat for termites depending on the type of building foundation. Avoid spraying chemicals. Treat the wood near the ground with boric acid while the framing is accessible. Sand and metal flashing inhibit termites. Sand under block or stone flooring may be treated with diatomaceous earth.

Finishing (Chapter 5: Remodeling)

Avoid carpeting. Hard wood floors, finished concrete, tile, cork, natural linoleum (manolium) are better choices. If you must have carpet, choose 100% wool with a felt backing. Don't put carpet in damp areas like bathrooms.

Buy kitchen cabinets constructed of either solid wood or exterior grade plywood. Avoid cabinets made with particleboard. Consider glass shelves or open cabinets with no doors.

Use zero-VOC paints and finishes.

Install a central vacuum cleaning system (Chapter 6: Dust)

Appliances (Chapter 7: Natural Gas)

Avoid gas and propane. On-demand, tank-less, electric water heaters are recommended.

If you must have gas, get a sealed combustion, power-vented system.

Room Layout (Chapter 8: Wiring)

Bedrooms should be at the furthest point from the fuse box.

Recreation, sitting, and office areas should be at least ten feet from the fuse box.

Appliances should not be on walls opposite bedrooms, especially where the head of the bed might be opposite an appliance or where people spend a lot of time sitting or children playing.

Install electrical wiring to minimize Electromagnetic Fields (Chapter 8: Wiring)

Use metal clad cabling or metal conduit to eliminate electric fields caused by house wiring.

Emphasize to the electrician the importance of not having any "net current" anywhere. Net current is against the National Electric Code (NEC) but common due to wiring errors. The most common wiring errors are ganging neutral wires from different branch circuits (one big wire-nut syndrome); and not using the correct wiring for 3-way switches.

Lighting (Chapter 8: Wiring)

Minimize fluorescent lighting, including compact-fluorescents. Compact fluorescents are being touted as environmentally-friendly because they save energy but they contain mercury and operate at a high frequency that gives some people headaches. Halogen lighting resembles natural light and is easier on the eyes. Halogens have transformers and should only be used for high ceilings above which there are no bedrooms.

Structure (Chapter 9: Mystery Toxins)

Build on a slab. Prior to pouring a slab, install a vapor barrier on top of coarse gravel. Do not put sand on top of a vapor barrier. It will trap moisture forever.

If there is a crawl space, make it a mini-basement by pouring a concrete slab and heating and ventilating it like a bedroom.

If the crawlspace won't have a slab, put a vapor barrier on top of the soil. Install perforated pipes and gravel under the vapor barrier with a fan to suck the moisture and odors out from under it similar to what is done for radon mitigation.

The garage should not to be connected to the house. Detached garages may be connected to the house by a breezeway. Don't put a garage under a bedroom.

Avoid fiberglass Insulation (Chapter 9: Mystery Toxins)

There are many alternatives types of insulation. For places where batt insulation is required, Bonded-Logic makes a cotton fiber batt insulation that is formaldehyde and fiberglass-free.

Post-Construction Clean-up (Chapter 9: Mystery Toxins)

Do not allow the furnace or air conditioning to be used during construction. Have it sealed up as soon as it's installed. If it is used ask the builder to clean the ductwork and furnace and change the filters before you move in.

Water

Order the 94-parameter water quality test kit from National Testing Laboratories, www.ntllabs.com or (800)458-3330. This will help you determine what kind of water filtration system is necessary.

If you are on city water, install a whole-house carbon filter to remove chlorine for showers and bathing.

Install a water filter under the kitchen sink for drinking and cooking. At a minimum you will to remove chlorine, lead, and dirt. Nearly all water filters sold remove these. If the city adds fluoride or there is arsenic or nitrates you will need a reverse-osmosis unit.

Heating and Air Conditioning system (Chapter: Furnace Filters)

Install a whole-house HEPA filtration system. Connect an outdoor air intake to it for fresh air.

Do not put ductwork or furnace cabinets in attics or crawlspaces. Do not allow the builder to use wall cavities for furnace air plenums. Seal every joint, seam, edge, and connection of the ductwork and furnace with mastic. Do not use duct tape. It will fall off.

SUGGESTED READING

A comprehensive *Guide to Building a Healthy Home* is available for free from the publisher of *Healthy Living Spaces: Top 10 Hazards Affecting Your Health.*

Send an email to FreeGuide@HealthyLivingSpaces.com

Baker-Laporte, Paula, Erica Elliot, M.D., and John Banta. *Prescriptions for a Healthy House. A Practical Guide for Architects, Builders & Homeowners.* New Society Publishers, 2001.

Johnston, David and Kim Master, *Green Remodeling, Changing the World One Room at a Time,* New Society Publishers, 2004.

The Architectural Resource Guide, edited by David Kibbey. An education directory of alternative building materials and suppliers. Order from the *Northern California Chapter of Architects, Designers and Planners for Social Responsibility.* Phone: (510) 845-1000. Email: admin@adpsr-norcal.org. Website: www.adpsr-norcal.org

Builder's Guide, Lstiburek, Joseph P.Eng., Energy Efficient Building Association. Phone: (952) 881-3048. Web site: www.buildingscience.com

END NOTES

1. Baker-Laporte, Paula and Robert Laporte. *Eco Nest. Creating sustainable Structures of Clay, Straw and Timber.* Gibbs Smith, Publisher, 2005, p. 40.
2. Robert Laporte is a timber framer and natural house builder. Paula Baker-Laporte is an architect specializing in healthy design. Their company, EcoNest™ works with clients to design their dream homes and teaches workshops in natural home building. Web site: www.econest.com. Phone: (505) 989-1813.

Tips for Creating a Healthier Bedroom

You spend a third of your life in the bedroom. The bedroom should be a place to rest and rejuvenate. The following are a few suggestions to make your bedroom a healthier living space:

Minimize the presence of electricity.

- Use a battery operated alarm clock.

- Remove as many electrical devices as possible from around the bed.

Get a Healthy Bed.

- Avoid metal. Metal frames and mattresses with springs cause localized magnetic fields that can be observed by placing a compass on top of the mattress and moving it around. Try a futon.

- Bedding and pillows should be made with natural or organic fibers such as cotton or wool.

Reduce the amount of plastic in the bedroom. Plastics deplete air of negative ions. Remove vinyl, synthetic fuzzy blankets, plastic lampshades, and plastic furniture.

Use non-fragrant laundry soap. One of the biggest exposures to chemicals is sheets and pillowcases that have been washed using fragranced laundry detergent and fabric softeners.

Minimize the presence of chemicals

- Do not use plug-in air fresheners.

- Do not use mothballs.

- Do not store dry-cleaned clothes in the bedroom closet.

Filter the air and let in some fresh air

- Get a HEPA air purifier. Turn it on high-speed an hour or so before you go to bed. You should be able to turn it down or off at night.

- Open the windows at night.

Layout for health

- The Chinese ancient art of Feng Shui suggests that bed be positioned diagonally opposite the door with the head of the bed away from it. This allows a view of the entry and control of one's destiny.

- Just moving the bed to a different location either in the same or a different room has alleviated symptoms of dis-ease and improved sleep for some individuals.

- Get rid of clutter that attracts and holds dust.

Select Bibliography

"Adverse Health Effects of Indoor Molds." *Journal of Nutrition and Environmental Medicine* (September 2004).

Anderson R.C., and J.H. Anderson. "Acute toxic effects of fragrance products." *Archives of Environmental Health* (March/April 1998).

Baker-Laporte, Paula, Erica Elliot, M.D., and John Banta. *Prescriptions for a Healthy House. A Practical Guide for Architects, Builders, & Homeowners.* Gabriola Island, British Columbia, Canada: New Society Publishers, 2001.

Bower, John. *The Healthy House.* Bloomington, IN: The Healthy House Institute, 1997.

Children's Health Environmental Coalition. *The Household Detective Primer, Protecting you children from toxins in the home.* Prinston, NJ: Children's Health Environmental Coalition, 2000.

Davis, Pamela J. "Molds, Toxic Molds, and Indoor Air Quality." California Sate Library: California Research Bureau, 2001.

Field Guide for the Determination of Biological Contaminants in Environmental Samples. Fairfax, VA: American Industrial Hygiene Association, 1996.

Gitterman, Heidi. "A Clear and Present Danger." *Alternative Medicine* (June 2002).

Gust, Lawrence. "Guidelines for Building a New Home." San Marcos, California: Lawrence J. Gust Consulting, copy obtained 2002.

Hansen, Shirley J., Ph.D. *Managing Indoor Air Quality.* Lilburn, GA: Fairmont Press, 1991.

Hollenden, Jeffrey. *Naturally Clean, The Seventh Generation Guide to Safe & Healthy Non-toxic Cleaning.* Gabriola Island, British Columbia, Canada: New Society Publishers, 2005.

IICRC S500 Standard and Reference Guide for Professional Water Damage Restoration, Second Edition. Vancouver, WA: Institute of Inspection, Cleaning, and Restoration Certification, 1999.

————. Vancouver, WA: Institute of Inspection, Cleaning, and Restoration Certification, 2003.

International Institute Bau-Biology and Ecology. Electro-Biology & Ecology and Air & Water, seminar notes. Clearwater, FL, 2001.

————. *Recommendations of Bau-Biological Standards Values.* Clearwater, FL, 1998.

Kail, Konrad, N.D., and Bobbi Lawrence. *Allergy Free, An Alternative Medicine Definitive Guide.* Tiburon, CA: AlterntiveMedicine.com, 2000.

Kosta, Louise A. *Fragrance and Health.* Atlanta, Georgia: The Human Ecology Action League, Inc., 1998.

Lankarge, Vivki. *What Every Home Owner Needs to Know about Mold (And What To Do About It).* Mc Graw Hill, 2003.

Lstiburek, Joseph, P., Eng. Builder's Guide, Hot-Dry and Mixed-Dry Climates. Minneapolis, MN: Energy Efficient Building Association, 1998.

Lynn Dadd, Debra. Home Safe Home, Protecting Yourself and Your Family from Everyday Toxics and Harmful Household Products. New York, NY: Penguin Putnam, 1997.

Macher, Janet, ed. *Bioaerosols: Assessment and Control.* Cincinnati, Ohio: American Conference of Governmental Industrial Hygienists, 1999.

May, Jeffrey C. *My House is Killing Me!* Baltimore, Maryland: The John Hopkins University Press, 2001.

May, Jeffrey C. and Connie L. *The Mold Survival Guide for your Home and for your Health.* Baltimore, Maryland: The John Hopkins University Press, 2004.

McAllister, Karen, BSc(hon), M.E.S., with assistance from Helen Lofgren, M.A. "Medical-Environment Report – A Review of the Potential Health Effects of the Proposed Sable Gas Pipeline Project from the perspective of Environmentally Induced Illness/Chemical Sensitivity, Asthma and allergy, prepared as part of an undertaking by the Allergy and Environmental Health Association." Nova Scotia: 1997.

Metro and the Oregon Department of Environmental Quality. Natural Gardening, A guide to alternatives to pesticides. Portland, OR: copy obtained 2004.

Miller, Norma L. Ed.D, ed. The Healthy School Handbook, Conquering the Sick Building S yndrome and Other Environmental Hazards in and Around Your School. Washington, D.C.: National Education Association (NEA), 1995.

Moses, Marion, M.D. *Designer Poisons, How to Protect Your Health and Home from Toxic Pesticides.* San Francisco, CA: Pesticide Education Center, 1995.

National Institute of Environmental Health Services and the U.S. Department of Energy. *Questions and Answers About EMF, Electric and Magnetic Fields Associated with the Use of Electric Power.* Washington, D.C.: U.S Government Printing Office, 1995.

New York City Department of Health. *Guidelines on Assessment and Remediation of Fungi in Indoor Environments.* New York, NY, 2002.

Olkowski, William. Common-Sense Pest Control. Newtown, CT: The Taunton Press, 1991.

Pearson, David. The New Natural House Book, Creating a Healthy, Harmonious, and Ecologically Sound Home. Fireside, 1998.

Pure Air Systems, Inc. Indoor Air Quality for the 21ˢᵗ Century, The Definitive Guide on Filtration, Ventilation and Environmental Control. Clayton, Indiana: Pure Air Systems Inc., 2002.

Riley, Karl. Tracing EMFs in Building wiring and grounding. Tucson, AZ: Magnetic Sciences International, 1995.

Spates, William. Various handouts provided during attendance of the Air, Water and Electro-Ecology seminars. Clearwater, Florida: Indoor Environmental Technologies, Environmental Testing and Consulting, 2001, 2002.

Sugarman, Ellen. Warning: the electricity around you may be hazardous to your health. Simon & Shuster, 1992.

Thompson, Athena. Homes that Heal (and those that don't); How your home may be harming your family's health. Gabriola Island, British Columbia, Canada: New Society Publishers, 2004.

United States Environmental Protection Agency. A Brief Guide to Mold, Moisture and Your Home. Washington, D.C., EPA 402-K-02-003.

———. Mold Remediation in Schools and Commercial Buildings. Washington, D.C., EPA 402-K-01-001.

———. The Inside Story, A Guide to Indoor Air Quality. Washington, D.C., 1995.

Wiles, Charlie. Certified Microbial Consultant (CMC) Review Course. Glendale, Arizona: The American Indoor Air Quality Council, 2003.

———. Strategies for Conducting Meaningful Microbial IAQ Investigations. Seminar. Glendale, Arizona: American Indoor Air Quality Council, 2002.

Wimberly, David. "Natural Gas: Avoidable Health Hazard." The Natural Gas Health Information Coalition, October, 2000.

Zamm, Alfred V., M.D. Why Your House May Endanger Your Health. New York, NY: Simon and Shuster, 1980.

A

acetone,
   in fragrance, 29
   in paint, 45, 43
active ingredients
   in cleaning supplies, 37
   in pesticides, 19, 22
AFM, 45, 46, 49
air conditioning, 2, 71, 75
   and mold growth, 7, 11, 71, 83
   and mystery toxins, 70
   and new construction, 94, 95
air fresheners, and fragrance, 20, 30-31, 98
air plenums, 70, 95
air filters and purifiers
   furnace, 52, 85-86
      antimicrobial coatings on, 84
      disposable, 85
      electronic, 82-84
      HEPA, 54, 72, 75, 84-86, 87, 95
      non-recommended, 82-84
      recommended, 85-86
      ultra-violet (UV) light as, 83
      washable, 82-83
   room, 86-88
      HEPA, 88, 98
      ionizers as, 84
      ozone as, 84, 87
      odor removal of, 88, 47
      non-recommended, 87
      recommended, 87
air purifiers: *see* air filters and purifiers
allergies: *see* health problems, allergies
American Indoor Air Quality Council, 16
ammonia, 33, 35, 40, 43

anti-bacterial: *see* anti-microbial
anti-microbials
   on air filters, 84
   in carpet, 46
   when furnace duct cleaning, 54
   in soap, 37-38
ants, getting rid of, 24-25
asbestos, 11, 16, 20, 51, 73, 84
Aspergillus mold, 84
asthma, *see* health problems, asthma
attics, 7, 61, 71, 95

B

bacteria, 37, 38, 71, 83, 84
bake-out, 47
baking soda, 32, 38
basements, 70, 71, 73, 94
bathrooms, 2, 29, 74, 92, 93
bedrooms, 7, 65, 66, 88, 93, 94, 97
bed-wetting, 65
beeswax, 39
benzene, 20, 22, 23, 29, 30, 38, 43, 44
biocides: *see* pesticides
bleach, 6, 10, 13, 17, 35, 37, 40-41
borax, 13, 32, 37, 39-39
boric acid, 24, 25, 93
breast cancer, 20, 22, 28
Bronner's soap, 13, 32, 37
Building Biology, v, 68

C

cancer, breast, 20, 22, 28
carbon monoxide, 58-59, 60, 61
car fumes, 43
carpet

chemicals emitted from, 33
deodorizing, 38
and dust, 52-53
health risks from, 43-44, 48
and mold growth, 12, 13
healthier alternatives to, 44, 49, 93
cats: *see* pet dander
ceilings
   and mystery toxins, 70, 72-73
   and wiring, 94
children
   and immune systems, 20
   and pesticide exposure, 21-22, 23
   and bed wetting, 65
chlorine bleach: *see* bleach
cleaning supplies, 35-42
   anti-microbials in, 37, 38
   choosing, 37
   disinfectants in: *see* anti-microbials
   health affects of, 36
   homemade, 38-39
   ingredients in, toxic, 35-36
Clorox: *see* bleach
cockroaches, 24, 51
cologne, 30, 32
compact fluorescent light bulbs, 94
concrete slabs, 49, 73, 93-94
condensation, 7, 47
crawl spaces, 70, 73-75, 94, 95

D

de-humidifiers, and air conditioning, 71
deodorizer blocks, 23
diatomaceous earth, 24, 93
dichlorobenzene: *see* mothballs

About the Author

Dan Stih is an aerospace engineer and environmental consultant who investigates homes and offices to solve complaints and health problems related to being indoors.

He got started in the business after retiring as an engineer from Motorola and taking up work as a handyman. While working as a handyman he discovered that some of his clients who were sick also had things wrong with the buildings they were living in. The buildings were responsible for their illness or making it difficult for them to be well again.

He lectures about how the indoor environment affects our health to anyone who will listen. For ongoing and updated information about indoor environmental issues, visit www.healthylivingspaces.com where you can sign up to receive Dan's free newsletter.

Dan currently lives in Santa Fe, New Mexico.

For Addition copies of:

Healthy LIVING SPACES

Top 10 Hazards Affecting Your Health

Daniel Stih, BSE, CMC, CIEC

Ask your local bookstore to order you a copy or visit our website at:
www.healthylivingspaces.com
or call 1(877) 992-9904

To order by Mail:
Enclose check with your order payable to
Healthy Living Spaces

(To the $18.95 cost per book, add $4.95 shipping for the first copy, and $1.50 for each additional copy).

For a free copy of the Mold Map™ – Levels of mold present in the state you live in, send an email to: MoldMap@HealthyLivingSpaces.com

Healthy Living Spaces

369 Montezuma Ave #169, Santa Fe, NM 87501
E-mail us at Orders@healthylivingspaces.com

There is a ton of information on HealthyLivingSpaces.com including chapters that did not make it into the final manuscript for *Healthy Living Spaces.*

Go to HealthyLivingSpaces.com to see it all.

Printed in the United States
85864LV00002B/1-249/A